CHOCOLATE CAKE IS THE BEST MEDICINE

THE BOND THAT TRIUMPHED OVER A NEAR-FATAL EQUINE ACCIDENT

Maria Duthie

Aurora Corialis Publishing
Pittsburgh, PA

Printed in the United States of America
Edited by Valentine Brkich, Aurora Corialis Publishing
Cover Design by Karen Captline, BetterBe Creative
Paperback ISBN: 978-1-958481-58-5
Ebook ISBN: 978-1-958481-59-2

Praise for Chocolate Cake

"*Chocolate Cake is the Best Medicine* tells the inspiring story of the author's journey overcoming significant vision impairment to lead a full life, fueled by her deep love for animals. Written in a clear, straightforward style, the book focuses on her near-fatal equestrian accident and her continued involvement in both equestrian and canine sports. Her story is deeply personal, offering a raw and touching glimpse into the challenges she faces and the resilience that drives her.

"The memoir also highlights her transformative trips to Africa, where she immerses herself in both the wildlife and culture of the countries she visits, adding another layer of richness to her narrative. For those who ride, participate in dog sports, or have faced personal adversity, this book offers powerful insights and inspiration. It's a must-read for anyone seeking a story of strength, determination, and overcoming life's obstacles. I highly recommend this book!"

Betsey Lynch
6x National Dog Agility Champion

"We are so grateful for Maria Duthie, our incredible equine massage therapist. Her ability to pinpoint exactly where each horse is sore or tight is truly remarkable. With her expert hands and deep understanding of performance horses, she keeps our five-star string feeling and moving their best. Maria is a vital part of our team, and we trust her completely to help keep our horses happy, healthy, and ready to perform at the highest level."

Rebekah Seger
Seger Sport Horses

"Find a cozy spot and prepare to meet one of the most fascinating people I know! This book gives us a glimpse into Maria Duthie's amazing world and her recovery from a terrible accident. She shares incredible stories of growing up riding horses, competing with agility dogs, and adventures in Africa, and she has been legally blind most of her life! Her pain is palpable as she retells her fateful accident and grueling recovery, describing moments of despair and small victories that kept her going. Whether you love animals like she does or stories about someone beating the odds, this book has something for everyone! You won't be able to put it down, and when you finish, you will be inspired to meet your next challenge head-on with grit and determination, just like Maria did."

Virginia Weida
Virginia Weida Designs LLC

"With each turn of the page, we can see that Maria has not been dealt the easiest hand in life, but what is abundantly clear is that she finds gratitude in every card she holds. Her perseverance and determination to keep showing up are genuinely inspiring. It seems as if she has lived many lives in this one lifetime, and she is thankful for what each has given her. *Chocolate Cake is the Best Medicine* is perfect for gaining perspective, encouraging gratitude, and inspiring readers to live life to the fullest."

Emily Hamel
International Five-Star Event Rider

"*Chocolate Cake* meets you directly in your heart. It speaks to the reader, calling out not only Maria's love for animals and her recovery from the accident, but also what she carried through her journey and what she will no longer keep buried. She names it. In full. Without apology.

"Maria isn't just telling a story with this book: she is showing you what it is to survive. She does so to change you, not to entertain you. This book is for those of us who had to choose between silence and survival. Who know what it's like to lose whole years to someone else's story. And now, what it's like after.

"Usually, we don't think about the 'after' part of our challenges. What comes beyond the healing. What life becomes. How that shifts. A huge percentage of trauma survivors don't thrive, but Maria shows us that thriving really is possible if we work toward what we want. I love that she focused on being able to ride again and used that to help her come back from the accident. It inspires us to push more so we can thrive too. What a beautiful story!"

Amanda Kunkle
Universe Liaison

"Maria Duthie shares deeply from her journey through life, from dealing with blindness at a young age to traveling around the world sharing her gift with animals. She is proof that it is not what happens to you in life that matters as much as your reaction to it. Maria's grace under pressure, hope and belief in a better day, and sheer grit and determination to make her many comebacks will serve as an inspiration to all. If you are seeking encouragement for your own challenges, are an animal lover, or a global citizen, this book is for you. Maria is the poster child of positivity."

Susan Hewitt, MA, LCMHC, SEP

"Maria's deep connection with animals, especially horses, shines through every page of her story. Her incredible journey of survival and recovery is a powerful reminder of how the love we share with animals can give us strength in our darkest moments."

Jennifer Crank
IncrediPAWS Dog Agility

Table of Contents

Note from the Pubisher

The following is the incredible true story of Maria Duthie and her survival and recovery from a near-fatal equestrian accident in July 2023. Maria became legally blind at a young age, and these struggles helped give her the fortitude to recover from the accident. The following story was compiled from journal entries transcribed from her dictated stories by her friend Virginia Weida.

"Life is either a daring adventure or nothing at all."
– Helen Keller

Introduction

Even though it's been two years, I still can't sleep sometimes because I keep thinking about it: The thing I love most of all nearly killed me that July morning.

I was literally minutes away from never waking up again. I thought I might never walk again. I drifted into unconsciousness and was no longer breathing. If I had moved even a little bit as I lay there, I would have been paralyzed, if not dead. Sometimes I wonder if it's just an illusion. Did I really die? But I'm still here. And somehow, I make strides every day, and I finally got back to doing what I love.

I survived Christopher Reeves' cervical vertebra number two break—the second bone away from the base of the skull. My vertebra was crushed into multiple pieces. There is no real explanation for why I survived, but I'm glad I did so I can share the story of my injury, my love for horses, and the inspiration that I hope it will be to others who think their dream has been taken away and need to work their way back to it again.

When the night is particularly still, it reminds me of the moment I almost stopped breathing, so I listen to sitcoms on my iPad at night to keep those thoughts away. Though the quiet is sometimes unsettling to me, it's also in these peaceful moments that I remember that this injury turned me into a fighter.

If you've gotten this far, then you're obviously someone who loves horses. If you ride, this book could be something that saves your life if you ever have an accident. Though the accident is the focus of this book, my whole life has prepared me for that day. Sometimes it takes a major tragedy to make you realize that you're stronger than you believed you were because you have been trained for the trials you will go through. Every hard day helps prepare us for the unknowns of the future so we can get through them and come out stronger on the other side.

Throughout my career working with animals and people, I realized that everyone goes through tough situations all the time, and I hope that my book can help you get through those times, leading with the same hope that I had that tomorrow will be a little easier, a little sweeter.

My hope for you is that you'll push through those challenges, and maybe there will be a little chocolate cake to celebrate, just like my horse, Chocolate Cake, has always been there for me.

Part One
Before

Legally Blind

You could tell from the time I was seven that something was wrong with my vision, but nobody could figure it out. I remember my brother Kevin holding a magazine up to me and saying, "Try to read this." He wasn't trying to be unkind; it was just that nobody understood. Thinking maybe I wasn't trying hard enough to see, I would work even harder. I was the kid who didn't want to be singled out. I didn't want attention, and I didn't want to be different. But, of course, those are the ones who end up being different, right? So, I tried to blend in as much as possible.

I first noticed something was wrong when I was in the first grade. We would do these math problems where you had to color parts of the page a certain color, but I always got it wrong because I was also colorblind. I always thought I was stupid. I remember crying because I could never get it right.

As I got older, I would try to hide it. I would make things up or pretend I could see when I couldn't. When I was ten, we went to the eye doctor, and he said I must be lying because there was no way I couldn't see like everyone else. When he'd leave the room, I'd run over to the eye chart, memorize it, and then return to the seat. You know how it is when you can sense that you're disappointing people, and I didn't want to disappoint anyone. After memorizing the chart, I'd get it right when the doctor returned. But, of course, when they changed the chart, the glasses they gave me didn't work.

My family moved from Whitefish Bay, Wisc., to Florida when I was a teenager, so I was able to go to the Bascom Palmer Eye Institute. That's when they finally diagnosed me with Stargardt disease. Stargardt's disease can't be diagnosed until the eyes mature, which is at thirteen years old. The doctors said my eyesight would continue to diminish throughout my life, and eventually, I would go blind. Not exactly what you want to hear. It wasn't a massive shock for us, though. I don't think it was a surprise to my mom and dad, either. They didn't treat me differently or act like I couldn't do anything. My mom was always super-supportive, and she was even planning to teach me how to drive if I wanted to learn, in case I ever had a situation where I needed to drive. They let me function as best as possible in society, which greatly helped me.

When I was diagnosed, I didn't have much training or resources to manage my disease. The school started providing some support, like occupational therapy, but that was merely a lady coming to show me how to use binoculars or magnifiers to read things. None of this made a huge difference in my life. I don't know if I was given all of the tools I could have been, or if I was not receptive to devices that would make me stand out.

I still enjoyed school, but I couldn't read things on the board. This was tough because I didn't want anyone to know I had an issue with my vision. It wasn't easy for me like it was for the other kids. Plus, I had to walk around with large-text books instead of normal ones. So, I stopped using all the tools they gave me pretty quickly because I wanted to fit in more. In high school, especially as a girl, it was more important not to be different than anything else. I think my vision issue affected my education and my career choices. If I'd had better support, things might've turned out differently. But, of course, nobody thought of those things then. I just felt like I didn't have any choice.

I can't say I didn't try as hard as I could in school. But I think I avoided facing the fact that I couldn't read certain things. Like I said, I wasn't given much support, other than being allowed to bring my dog to school. Looking back, I think my life would've been much different if I had normal vision, but it probably wouldn't have been as much fun. For example, I might not have gone on as many trips or been as adventurous as I have been. In a way, it's been a blessing.

My Lifelong Love of Animals

My early years were interesting. I was adopted at three months of age, which never really bothered me. I've known my whole life that I was adopted, and I've always known that my parents had "chosen" me. I was the youngest in a family of four, with a sister who was twelve years older, two teenage brothers dealing with their own issues, and a father who was actively drinking throughout most of my youth.

Mom and I, however, could not have been any closer. I adored her as a child and would follow her everywhere. I would watch her (more like spy on her; it was probably a little creepy), but I thought she was the best thing on earth. I don't know why I was so attached to her. She always said that we had been together in another life, and the story continues to be true.

I have been obsessed with horses since the time I could walk. When I was two, my parents put me on a horse alone. I rode that horse on a trail ride, with a lady leading on her horse, but she didn't hold mine at all. I was on him all by myself. After that, I was hooked, and I spent every bit of money I had on rides at fairs and carnivals. My friend Julie and I even made TV stands into horses so we could pretend to be riding. All of my Christmas lists started like this: horse, pony, stuffed animal horse, dog, puppy, and anything *horse*.

My first job was as a trail guide when I was nine, and it always made me feel so cool. I had a crush on Chuck, who taught me to ride bareback. One day, I remember riding bareback up to our trailer at a place we'd go to in the summers. As I did, my brother, Mom, and the others came out to see me, and they were so impressed. On those trails, riding those horses, I felt so powerful and confident, like I could do anything. We'd race down the dirt road, and it was so much fun. I was actually good at it! The horses gave me freedom and confidence.

When I turned thirteen, we left that place and moved down to Florida. It was a big change for me and a difficult one. But then I got my first horse, Kristi. I also worked at a farm, riding the trails and tacking up horses for people to ride on their own around the property. We'd ride the trails, too, just to make sure they were okay. It was another fun job where I met my first boyfriend. I enjoyed being there, out on the farm, having mud fights, and riding horses. I mean, what could be better?

During college, I worked at the University of Florida's poultry farm, which was a nightmare. But I didn't have much money then, so I had no choice. I did enjoy parts of it, though, because I was on a farm. I liked the research side of things, but I didn't like the processing side. However, since I didn't have much money, it was a good way to get food. And let me tell you, I ate a lot of eggs!

After college, I worked as a zookeeper in Indianapolis for four and a half years. The job was great, but like the poultry farm, it paid nothing, which was frustrating at times. But then I gave two presentations at the American Association of Zookeepers convention and became involved in fundraising and behavioral enrichment projects. That became my main focus. Unfortunately, I eventually had to leave that job because of my vision loss.

I started searching for something new. When I was working at a barn driving ponies, I discovered animal massage, which would become my primary career for the next twenty-eight years. I was determined to make enough money to care for my horses and was much more successful than I ever imagined I could be. Through this occupation, I've been able to travel worldwide, working on dogs and horses, and also teaching. I've also met many people and traveled all over the country with my dog, Flip, who was my heart and soul. I love giving something back to the animals that have given so much to me. I love watching their relationships with their owners and then helping the owners take even better care of them.

We moved from Ohio to Aiken, South Carolina, in 2022 because of the horses and the weather. We moved into a horse community so I could get to trails without being dependent on someone to drive me. In a horse community, if I need help, I always have someone around. Life in Aiken is different. I am grateful for the opportunity to be here. We often go out to dinner with friends, and we get to enjoy live music in the alley, where you can bring your dog, hang out, and just walk around. We love that. I ride a lot with friends and have fantastic trainers for my horses. Well, I should say, for me, when I'm riding my horses. It's kind of like living in a fantasy. Our neighborhood's speed limit is twenty-five, and you barely hear any traffic. I look out my bedroom window, and all I see are trees. It's all trees outside the sliding glass door in the living room and the kitchen window. In the winter, you can hear whippoorwills at night. It's a horse-focused community, which has been wonderful in many ways.

A typical day for me in Aiken starts with waking up and walking the dogs on the trails in the neighborhood. When I come home, I bring in the horses, feed them, and then work in my arena, the public arena, or on the trails, either by myself or with a friend. Then, I'll swim in the pool, take another walk, feed the horses, and go out to dinner. Soon after that, I'm off to bed. Sometimes, we ride in Hitchcock Woods, which is amazing, and sometimes we bring the horses to the Wilcox, sit outside with them, and have lunch and a cocktail. It's a slice of life that doesn't exist in many places, and I'm lucky to enjoy it.

My love of animals brought me to a special community. It gave me a level of confidence that people with normal vision might take for granted. When you enter a space where you don't know anything, having an animal with you, especially riding a horse, is like having an extra set of eyes. Working with animals has given me a sense of freedom I wouldn't have had without it.

Riding Lessons

Despite my vision challenges, I accomplished a lot of things by showing horses. I think my love of riding and showing horses grew because I had experienced many early successes. I'm sure that's true for everyone. But for me, it made the playing field feel more even. I was good at riding and comfortable on horses, which proved I could do things like others. I trust the horses I ride, and it helps when you have the right one.

Growing up riding, I was successful on the local level and somewhat on the circuit level. I did some eventing with one horse, which was a lot of fun. And I did well. At least, that is until I didn't. When I moved up to higher levels, it became too difficult to see where I was going on the course, which made it much more challenging and unfair to the horse. So, we stayed at a certain level. So, I got more into hunter-jumpers, because the courses are right there, and you can look at them beforehand.

To compensate for my visual issues, I sometimes took pictures of the ring. My trainers would then have me walk around the ring so I could see the different angles of the jumps. I'd do these walks early in the morning, just to get an idea of where to turn. Over time, this has gotten a little easier for me to manage. Looking straight ahead is kind of easy, as long as you roughly know where the turn or jump is. I'm not saying I've never missed a jump— because I have! But it's not too bad if you can just memorize where you're going.

The first special horse in my life was Kiowa, a brown and white American Paint Horse I rode during my first job on the trails when I was nine. I was shy as a kid—really shy—and I didn't like to talk or make too much noise. I didn't feel special at all, and I just wanted to be out of the picture. But when I would ride Kiowa, I felt like I could do anything. Whether it was racing through the barn and grabbing the rafters to swing like a fool or learning to ride bareback for the first time, I felt so free. Whenever we'd go to

Rubidell, the trailer park we visited every summer for vacation, I finally felt special. That's because my brothers weren't riding bareback like I was, and they couldn't go as fast as I could. I could get Kiowa to do things they couldn't.

Rubidell is also where I had my first crush: Chuck. Chuck taught me to ride bareback. He was probably seventeen or eighteen at the time, and he was always so nice. Eventually, he went off and joined the army. I don't know what happened to him after that, but I hope he grew up to have an amazing, happy life, with a wife, kids, and horses, of course.

If I'm being honest, Kiowa wasn't technically my first *special* horse. I guess my first truly special horse was when I was two. As I mentioned earlier, my mom's friend put me on her daughter's horse by myself, and she didn't lead me or have another horse guide me. The two of us went on a trail ride that lasted about half an hour to an hour. I was a nervous wreck at first, but once I started riding, I was a natural.

A couple of years later, my mom's friend's daughter had a tragic accident when she was riding a horse that threw her into a telephone pole. She was killed. But that didn't make me want to stop riding. In fact, I was more concerned about what happened to the horse. I asked my mom what they did with it, and she told me they sold the horse, which made me sad.

My second special horse was a pony we found on the side of the road. We were driving through the mountains in upstate New York, on our way to Ryder Lake to visit my grandparents. The roads were winding and narrow, and as we turned a corner, we spotted a pony on the side of the road. My mom turned to me and said, "Maria, can you get out and get that pony?" So, I did. I grabbed our dog Tiger's leash, put it over the pony's neck, and walked it down the road all by myself, with the car and the family following behind. We eventually found where the pony lived. You can imagine what a boost of confidence it gave me, an awkward, visually impaired seven-year-old, to be out on my own with that beautiful little pony.

Then came my *very special* horse, Kristi, a blood bay mare with a white star, an Anglo-Arabian. I started riding her during my lessons when we moved to Florida. I was riding Western style at first, but I didn't care much about the discipline. My mom wanted me to learn English-style riding, so she enrolled me in lessons at B-Bar-B Stables in Fort Lauderdale. A woman named Sue Hurley provided the lessons, which I did while riding Kristi. I fell madly in love with Kristi, especially when I found out she was for sale. I wanted to keep that horse more than anything.

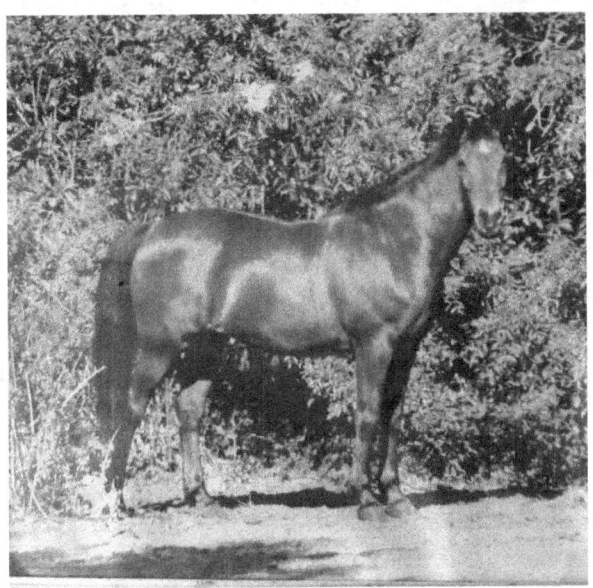

You see, we had moved to Florida on my thirteenth birthday from Whitefish Bay, Wisc. This was a huge culture shock for me, and therefore, I really, really wanted that horse. My parents had friends in town one night, and we all went out for dinner. There, they all gave me a hard time about how I would never get that horse. I got really upset at this, left the restaurant, and walked home.

But then my mom took me to my next lesson, and at the end of the lesson, Sue turned to me and said, "Okay, you can go ahead and do whatever you want," adding, "Kristi is yours. Your parents bought her for you." I felt like I grew ten feet right there. I was standing there with Kristi—my horse—and it was incredible. After that, I went into the field, rode around on her, brushed her, and cared for her. Choosing where I wanted to go and how fast I wanted to go was an amazing feeling. I guess it's like how people feel when they get their first car.

I did everything with Kristi. We showed; we jumped. Sometimes, I would line up the day campers and jump them (probably not the safest thing in the world, but it was fun!). Later, I taught her to rear and rode her in my high school's homecoming parade. Eventually, I took her to college. Later, I took her to Canada with me when I got married.

I just loved being with Kristi, even if that was just spending time with her in the barn. Before we got married, I told my husband, Ken, that there was nowhere I'd rather be than in the barn with Kristi. But our special bond would end too soon. Tragically, one day, a man with a severe heart condition hit and killed Kristi on the side of the road while I was riding her. Losing Kristi the way I did was very difficult.

I took her for a ride that day with my dog Rusty at my side. At the time, we were living in a very rural area of Canada, and we were going down the dirt road heading over to some trails that I really enjoyed riding. Our neighbor came driving by; we were probably two farms down from home. I heard him coming and pulled way over to the right, and he still hit us. Apparently, he was on heart medication that was making him really unfit to drive.

I woke up probably 30 feet from her in the middle of the road. I don't remember much, but I remember hitting the hood of his car. Nobody was around when I woke up except for my dog. Rusty sat beside me. I got up and went over to Kristi. My beautiful horse lay dying on the road with a broken femur after we were hit. It was horrific. I couldn't help but stand there, watching her, trying to figure out what to do. I didn't have a phone. I just started screaming for help. I sat with her, hugged her, and did my best to keep her calm. She deserved way more than that tragic ending to her life. She was with me through all of my growing-up years, through the bad times and the good times, my constant friend and companion.

Because of the way I lost her, it made me want to learn to do something, anything. No massage would have healed my horse, but it would have made her more comfortable and relaxed, so that's what I chose to do. I tried to make one good thing come out of that horrendous day when my heart was broken as I lost my best friend.

Following the accident, I was tortured by thoughts of *Did I do the right thing? Did I make a mistake? Could I have saved her? Is there anything else I could've done?* I even made multiple phone calls to the vet, asking if there was anything more I could have done. I don't wish that pain on anyone, but I do hope everyone has a relationship as beautiful and pure as mine and Kristi's because she was such a great horse and taught me so much. It nourished my love of horses to this day, and I am grateful to have known her. This tragic end to her life did not dampen my love for horses.

When I really think about it, all of my horses have been special and provided me with different things. Dylan, for example, was my first eventing horse. River was a low-level hunter jumper that I broke and trained myself to ride. Penzi, which means "love" in Swahili, was the first horse I received as a gift on my birthday, and she was just the most fun and willing horse ever.

And then, of course, there's Chocolate Cake. Chocolate Cake was my first warmblood. I got her when she was fourteen months old after I'd lost my beloved Jessie. Now that I think about it, Jessie—a quarter horse filly that I bought in college—was my actual first baby and the first that I broke and trained on my own to ride. I had been planning to train and sell her, but that never happened. I kept telling my mom, "There are just a few more things I need to teach her first."

Jessie passed away from cancer at my farm in Medina, Ohio. When I lost her to cancer, I was devastated. But from that, I got Chocolate Cake, my best hunter-jumper horse, who took me on a new learning curve. She is my derby and adult amateur horse. Chocolate Cake is fun, super-athletic, and willing to jump over anything. I placed 8th in the Ohio Derby Series one year with her, and she also showed a lot in adult amateur classes, doing quite well for me.

I enjoyed the derby series because I could walk the course. This allowed me to find all the fences, and walk all the turns, which gave me a lot of confidence jumping the course, similar to dog agility. Cake was the first horse on which I was able to jump tall fences. The highest I ever jumped her was 3'9". She showed in the adult amateur division at 3' and in the derby with 3'5" options. Cake definitely took me to a different level in showing and boosted my confidence.

One July day, we were showing at Chagrin in the adult amateurs. But as we cantered up to the fence to jump down a line, she just stopped. Cake just crumbled. It was like she was exhausted, and it felt like she couldn't possibly lift herself off the ground, let alone over the fence. She had been acting strangely all day and wasn't very happy, which was disappointing because it should have been easy for her. She had been to that venue a million times before.

The vet couldn't find anything wrong, so we went to another show and had a professional ride her to see if it would make a difference, but it didn't. Once again, Cake crumbled in front of the fence. I had my farrier look at her, and she said there was something wrong with her shoe. So I was like *Oh well, this must be the problem*, but it wasn't. I should've known when it happened the first time and certainly when it happened the second time that this horse was injured.

It broke my heart trying to figure out what was going on with her. She would get a little better and then backslide. Finally, they determined that injecting her sacrum would make a difference. I wasn't convinced that was the situation, but I thought maybe it would help. She had a lot of swelling and inflammation in her quadriceps that we could see with ultrasound. She showed lameness on the front and not much behind. I had a lot of gait analysis, special shoeing, and injections done. In the end, none of it helped. In fact, the injections actually made it worse because they only masked the pain, and she did too much because she couldn't feel it.

I had moved down to Aiken, S.C., near my trainer's facility. I was there at the facility one day when, suddenly, during a lesson, Chocolate Cake came up lame on her front left leg. My trainer then referred me to Dr. Peroni out of Athens, Ga. Thank goodness for my trainer, Rebekah Seger, who was friends with Doug Payne. Doug had two horses that had undergone surgery on their stifles at the University of Georgia in Athens. So I took Cake to Athens, where Dr. Peroni performed surgery on her in January of 2023. By the time Chocolate Cake had the surgery, her patella tendon was nearly torn through! The vet was able to burn the tissue to create more scar tissue. We also did stem cells. If I had not done the surgery, I would not have had very many options; certainly none for recovery. That experience was terrifying. I'd had Chocolate Cake since she was eighteen months old, and we're as close as a person and horse can be. Truly, she's my friend. She's taken me places I thought I'd never go.

After Cake's surgery, we started the rehabilitation process. I was grateful to be an animal massage therapist, which allowed me to work on all of her muscles. I'd been an equine and canine masseuse for years. It's one of the few jobs I can do while being visually impaired. I used laser therapy daily on Chocolate Cake and hand-walked her, doing everything she needed to get better. It was a slow process, but it was going well. Eventually, she was turned out in a small paddock, then into a bigger one, and finally out into the pasture. It was amazing, and it felt great. I could then start walking and trotting with her. Soon, I began cantering. It was amazing to see her healthy and getting ready to jump over the cross rails. I was very happy with the outcome; however, she was delayed in her rehab because of my accident. I never imagined that we would be in recovery together, which brought us even closer.

Strength in Stillness

My accident in 2023 was not my first serious spinal injury; I broke my back when I was ten years old, jumping out of a second-story window in an old duplex in Whitefish Bay, Wisc. Julie, another girl, and I were in a bedroom at the time, and we were bored. So, we decided we'd climb out of the window using a jump rope. I must've psychically known I would be using my hands in my career, so as I climbed down the rope, which was rough and frayed, I let go of it and fell to the ground. My friend Julie was already down there, and she was screaming bloody murder. "Come on!" she said. "Get up! You're going to be okay!" But I couldn't get up. I couldn't stand. It hurt too much, so I didn't even try.

Julie immediately ran off and got my mom, who called 911. When I arrived at the emergency room, the orthopedist examined me and then asked me, "Do you ever want to ride horses again?" I told him, "Yes, of course!" And he replied, "Then you will not move one muscle." So I didn't. I just lay there in my bed, trying to be still, for two long weeks. For a ten-year-old, this wasn't easy. I don't remember much about it, but I think I had a brace on and had to lie flat. It was awful. It was not particularly painful, but it was still miserable and uncomfortable.

During my recovery, there were a couple of funny things that happened. First, my friend Heather came to visit me. She, too, was just ten, but for some reason, she was allowed to take me downstairs to get some fresh air in the hospital's little garden area. They actually let a ten-year-old wheel another ten-year-old down the elevator and out the front doors. Probably not the best idea. There was a hill outside the hospital, and Heather rolled me down it on the gurney. Then, she lost control and let go. Amazingly, it sailed perfectly flat, with me never moving a muscle, into the parking lot, right where my dad was pulling in to visit. From that point on, they called me the "Flying Nun."

Another funny thing was when my sister and her then-boyfriend pushed me up the parking garage ramp, all the way to the top, so I could watch the fireworks, lying flat on my back. They also brought my dog, Tiger, to see me, but I could only see him while I was outside. Again, I never moved the entire time. I'd just lie there and watch him play in the parking lot while I remained perfectly still.

Nights were probably the worst. I'd spent so much time away from home, and I was scared and lonely. But, eventually, it all worked out. I distinctly remember the day I was allowed to walk for the first time. I didn't think it would be a big deal. After they put a brace on me, they stood me up, and I walked across the room. Immediately, Julie and my parents started clapping. I guess there was some question if I would ever walk again. They should've just asked me!

Another experience that probably helped prepare me for my accident as an adult happened at a trailer in Wisconsin near the Crawfish River, where we sometimes went on the weekends. During one of these weekends, a teenage boy had been swimming in the river off the boat launch, broke his neck, and was paralyzed. I remember my mom saying that you must remain still when you break your back. That advice stuck with me, and I think it helped me stay calm during my injury.

Service Dogs to Agility Champions

I started dog agility after I began massaging dogs. It looked fun, and I wanted to understand what the dogs and handlers were going through. Agility courses have maps, and the handlers have to follow a numbered course with their dogs. You may be wondering how I learn the courses with my visual impairment. In the beginning, they would print out large paper maps for me to use, especially at national-level competitions. But now, with maps being sent out electronically, I blow them up on my phone to review, and most often, I just follow other handlers when walking the courses.

The first dog I worked with on agility was a rescue named Bailey. She's the one I wish I could do over again. Being my first dog, I made a lot of mistakes. She was stressed, and we just didn't have a good connection. She was fast and fun, but we couldn't gel as a team. We did make it to the "excellent" level, though.

The next dog was Flip, the foundation sire I've used for all of my dogs since then. Flip wasn't the fastest or the best agility dog. Initially, he too was stressed out and would walk the course without wanting to do anything. The weave poles were a nightmare. I told him, "If you don't want to do this anymore, just sit on the course tomorrow and don't move. I don't care if you run around like a fool, but if you don't want to do it, just sit there." From that day forward, we got past our stress, and Flip ran around like a fool. I showed him at the USDA Nationals in Arizona, and it was just so much fun.

Flip went through a battle with lymphoma when he was two, but he lived until he was almost fourteen. When he was six, he fell out of the hayloft and broke his elbow. Flip was my first service dog, and he and I traveled nationwide together, teaching massage seminars. He was the father of Spin and Tumble, my most successful agility dogs. They were littermates though they looked nothing alike.

Spin and Tumble gave me my first MACH (Master Agility Champion) titles. By the end of their careers, Spin and Tumble each had six MACHs. Tumble also had one PACH, and Flip had two PACHs. All three dogs went to the USDA, AKC Nationals, CPE Nationals, and UKI US Open. Tumble and Spin were on the podium at the UKI US Open. The first year, sadly, I didn't realize Tumble had placed after all, and I left before I got the chance to be on the podium, so I had to photoshop myself and Tumble into the podium picture!

We returned to the UKI US Open the following year, however, where Spin won the biathlon and Tumble placed in games and the national finals. I was very proud of those boys and enjoyed them so much. They were always back-to-back on the Nationals list because they were as fast as I was. They were just great dogs and a lot of fun.

The first time I took all three dogs to the AKC Nationals in Reno was an unforgettable experience. I had Flip, Spin, and Tumble with me, and they were full of energy. When we were warming up for a run, Spin jumped up toward my face and hit me in the eye with his nose, so I ended up with a black eye. Later, when I was exercising them outside, Tumble knocked me over, kind of like a football player tackling me, and I landed on my back. After that, I had to trade with a massage therapist for some bodywork for me. They were just full of energy—fun, fun, fun dogs! I'm so grateful to have had them. They gave me so much success and confidence in my agility career.

I also ran a dog named Slide, but he isn't much of a team player. He is very fast, but he wouldn't tolerate any handling mistakes. As he got older, he became more stressed in the ring, and I didn't want any incidents that might make him seem aggressive. In the end, he became my home agility dog. He is the fastest dog I've ever had—so talented—but he didn't enjoy showing like my other dogs do.

Then there's Zigzag, Flip's grandson and Tumble's son, who loves agility more than life itself. He reminds me a lot of Spin and

Tumble. Spin loved the sport; Tumble just did it for the food (he loved agility, but food was his ultimate reward). Zigzag is a bit more of a puzzle to figure out, but not in the same way as Slide was. He's much more forgiving and allows me to make mistakes as long as we're on the same page. And when we are, we have some beautiful, fast runs together. Zigzag loves the sport so much that just doing it is his reward.

Zigzag excels in every sport he tries. He's a multi-talented dog, much like his grandfather, Flip. He has titles in Barn Hunt, Lure Coursing, Dock Diving, Scent Work, Rally, and Agility, of course. All of my dogs have earned multiple titles in various venues and disciplines, and Zigzag is no exception.

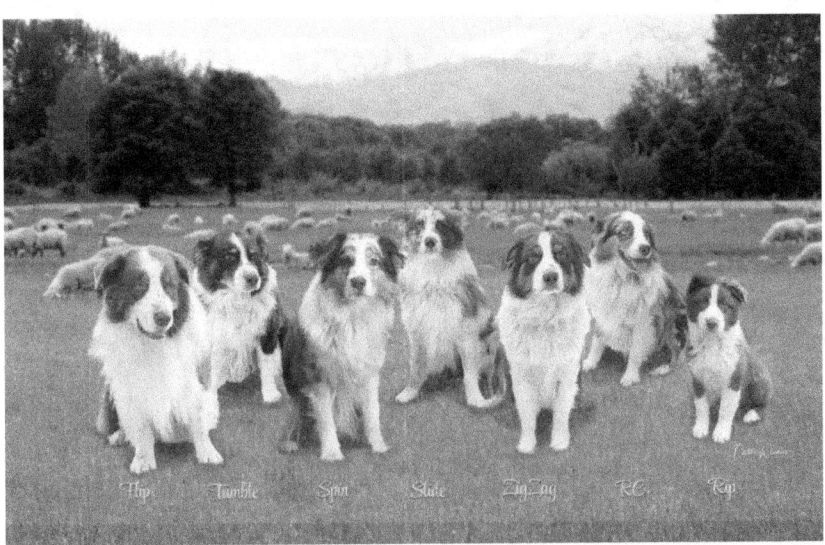

Then there's Rip, my youngest dog. Rip isn't the fastest agility dog, though he has a lot of speed; he prefers to use it for games rather than work. He's very accurate and has actually earned more double Qs (i.e., earning qualifying scores in both the Master Standard and Master Jumpers With Weaves classes on the same day at the same trial) than Zigzag at this point. Rip doesn't often make mistakes. Occasionally, he'll take an off-course tunnel, but for the most part, he's very focused. He's still learning the full value of agility, but for him, praise and food are his biggest motivators. He's a funny, talented little dog, and I know he'll be successful. We've taken our time working together, building confidence, and making sure he understands the rewards for his efforts. Rip has already shown at the U.S. Open alongside Zigzag, and I'm excited to see what his future holds.

I competed at national events from Florida to California in dog agility, and likewise, I have also had the opportunity to travel nationally and internationally with US Agility teams to massage dogs in Austria, Germany, and Belgium. Seeing the faster and most finely tuned dog-and-handler teams worldwide has been a wonderful opportunity. It is a huge honor and lots of fun whenever I can participate. Being a minor contributing factor to the team's success is terrific.

Adventures in Africa

My first trip to Africa was like a dream come true. I had always wanted to go, and when the opportunity came, I was beyond excited. A friend I had made before it was impossible for me to continue as a zookeeper won a trip to Kenya. She and I went over together for *Bowling for Rhinos*, a fundraiser for the Lewa Downs Animal Sanctuary, and we were treated like royalty.

I did some crazy things while in Africa, like sleeping outside on couches in the middle of the wilderness, with leopards roaming nearby. One night, we turned on a flashlight and discovered a black female rhino just ten feet away, which was incredible. The stars in the African sky were like nothing I had ever seen. They were so bright and close, it felt like you could reach out and touch them.

We had all kinds of exciting adventures on that trip. We got a flat tire in the middle of a field full of white rhinos. Another time, we were charged by a black rhino that was breeding. We also had a close encounter with an elephant in musk. Another one of the highlights was horseback riding. It was incredible to be out there on horseback, riding through the wild, getting so close to giraffes and zebras. It was a perspective I had never experienced before, and it made everything feel even more alive. Being in the vast, open space with all that wildlife and freedom was the most fantastic feeling.

For me, it was also an opportunity to test my vision. I wanted to see just how far I could push myself in terms of what I could see, so I kept trying to look farther and farther into the distance. That trip allowed me to challenge myself and see how much I could experience.

While in Africa, I also shared that I was an animal massage therapist. To my delight, I was invited back a few more times to work on horses and orphaned wildlife at Lewa Downs Sanctuary. On one of my visits, I spent hours working with their horses and even had the opportunity to teach the Maasai how to massage them. I learned some Swahili to teach them properly, and it was a rewarding experience. Later, they told me how they had used the massage techniques I showed them, not just on their horses, but also on each other and their cattle.

It was such an incredible experience to be able to give back in that way, teaching something that had been so valuable to me and seeing how those people integrated it into their daily lives. It was also amazing to work with their horses and help train them. That trip is something I will never forget.

During my time in Africa, I had the privilege of working with orphaned wildlife, which added another layer to my incredible journey. One of the most memorable massages I performed was for an orphaned black rhino named Omni. I had watched Omni when he was just six months old, and by the time I saw him again at two years old, I was able to massage him. Omni let me know when he was done with the massage in the best way possible—he picked up a log and chased me around with it!

I worked with kudu, cheetah cubs, and some polo ponies. These animals were such a joy to work with, and I felt fortunate to be able to help them in any way I could. But what I received in return was even greater than what I gave. Each experience was deeply rewarding. One of my favorite memories was watching three cheetahs hunt as a pack. That's not typical cheetah behavior, as they usually hunt alone, but these were special. They had even managed to take down a giraffe together—again, not something you typically see cheetahs do.

I also had the incredible opportunity to see a baby giraffe just moments after it was born. That was truly a once-in-a-lifetime experience. I encountered old buffalo resting in caves, huge tire-sized tracks from a boa constrictor (though I can't be sure if it was actually a constrictor), and so much more. Another of my favorite activities was lion tracking. It was such a fantastic experience until I realized that the sound of my camera rewinding didn't sit well with the lions. I nearly got into trouble for that one!

Another unforgettable experience was going on a zebra knockdown project, where we documented stripe patterns to determine individual differences. It was fascinating. While they were sedated, I had the chance to massage the zebras' muscles and get a closer feel for their anatomy.

On my first trip to Africa, I went for the animals but ended up falling in love with the people. The kindness, intelligence, and generosity I encountered were truly humbling. I can't say enough about the friends I made there. My heart definitely belongs to Kenya.

I actually went to a Maasai wedding on my second trip. We went to the village before the wedding, and the warrior getting married had a George W. Bush sign and a Bush bumper sticker on his hut. We thought that was pretty funny. When we went to the wedding, the children had never seen white people before! The bride was thirteen. They loaded a trunk with her belongings and dowry and walked over the hillside. She's not allowed to look back to say goodbye, and that child will never see her family again. They received gifts of goats and things like that. It's the way they live. After the wedding, we walked back along the riverbed, and some Maasai warriors had just killed the goat. They offered us some goat meat, so we ate barely cooked goat over an open fire with four amazing young men I will never forget.

One of my most humbling experiences during my third or fourth trip to Kenya was visiting a local school with school supplies and donations. When the children arrived, they were orderly, neatly dressed, and respectful. Despite having so little, they greeted us with songs and big smiles, acting like proper ladies and gentlemen. The respect they showed us was deeply moving.

Afterward, the teachers and the principal invited us to stay for a meal. They served us maize and sweet potato cooked in river water—the same water they had used to wash our hands before we ate. It was a simple meal, but one that was made with so much love and generosity. Their hospitality was overwhelming, and I felt so blessed to be there.

The next day, I became very ill, likely from the food, but I couldn't bring myself to resent their kindness. Even though I was sick, I knew that refusing their gift would have been disrespectful. So, I ate their meal with gratitude because it symbolized their warmth and culture, and the humility they displayed while welcoming us into their world.

The people I met in Kenya don't expect anything. They are grateful for everything, no matter how little they have. From that experience, I ran a nonprofit for a few years, which helped fund schooling for children there, sending kids to school and even to college, which felt very meaningful to me.

One of the most memorable parts of my time there was walking every day at lunch with my friend Patrick. Because of the wildlife, I couldn't walk alone, so Patrick, one of the dancers we'd seen in the bush, would accompany me.

Seeing the Maasai dancers perform was one of the most incredible things I've ever witnessed. They leaped so high in the air; their athleticism is unbelievable. As we walked, we chatted about the dance, and I made a deal with Patrick: I would teach him to waltz if he would teach me how to dance like a Maasai. So, there we were, waltzing along through the African prairie. The English owners of the reserve drove by, and I'm sure they didn't quite understand the bond we were forming. The Maasai and the English had very different relationships with the land, but Patrick and I were friends, no matter our differences.

One day at lunch, Patrick and I came across a dead zebra with marks on its side. We immediately informed the conservationists, who took us to the field with them. There, we learned that a lion had attacked the zebra. She'd been able to run away but had eventually died of internal bleeding. Her baby only lasted the night before the predators got to him, too. We returned later that evening, hoping to see what had happened to the zebra. We brought a leg of the zebra with us, which we gave to a leopard waiting in a tree.

When we returned to check on the zebra's carcass, hyenas were everywhere. There wasn't a trace of the zebra left. This was a haunting but natural process and a reminder of how animals depend on each other in a delicate system of life and death. The next day, I saw another zebra, which was smaller—perhaps a young one—still with its mother. Seeing the animals interact like that was a powerful reminder of the interconnectedness of everything.

That trip helped me understand the deep system of respect that exists between the Maasai, the wildlife, and the land. I grew to love and admire this way of life immensely, which honors all things, from the smallest plant to the largest predator.

On my fourth trip, a nurse volunteered with me, and we were invited to attend a local church service. It turned out to be one of the most amazing experiences of my life. The people there came dressed in suits, which had obviously been donated from Europe and the United States. I remember one rail-thin man, whose gray suit hung loosely on him. He looked at us and said, "God bless you. We will pray for you." The humility and grace with which they expressed their gratitude for the smallest things was overwhelming. They wanted to give, love, and bless us, without expecting anything in return. That moment, that gesture, really changed me. It made me realize that giving doesn't always come with expectations—it can come from pure, selfless kindness.

Another memorable experience during that trip was going to an AIDS orphanage, where I videotaped Irene leaning against a small metal hut. She was wearing ragged clothes and looked bad. She looked very tired, like she needed to be in bed. Irene had a sack of groceries that she had gone to the store to get. She told us the story of how Somali rebels had come down across the border, which was very close, raped her daughter and son, who both ended up dying of AIDS, and raped her, too. I believe they killed her husband, as well. Now, she sat just outside of that AIDS orphanage, waiting to die.

They didn't have treatment like they could've gotten here. When we walked through the orphanage, all these children had AIDS, and the only medication they could give them was not going to cure them or prolong their lives like we could do for them. They only had a few sacks of grain piled up in an empty storeroom to feed all these people. I'll never forget the one little girl with bright eyes and a big smile. It haunts me to this day that she didn't get the treatment she deserved. When you see things like that, it changes you forever in a good way. I am so grateful to all of them for the opportunities they've given me to see things from another side.

Things like this are difficult to see, but they and all the natural beauty are what make Africa special. These people keep going and are grateful for each day, whether they are orphans, dying, or helping those who are. Their strength is like that of the amazing animals that surround them.

Wild Expeditions

My trip to Uganda, Kenya, and Rwanda in January 2007 was amazing and life-changing. It was filled with amazing animals and unforgettable people. We saw everything from refugee camps in Uganda to wealthy people trying to make a difference in these fantastic countries.

Both Uganda and Rwanda were very safe. We could walk around with no problems in every city we went to. In Kabale, Uganda, I bought some peas from a little girl to give her something. I decided to leave them because they needed them more than I did, but they ran after our tour guide to ensure I got them back. The peas traveled to Rwanda, where we gave them, along with any other leftover food, to our gorilla guide, Francis. The night before our trek to see the gorillas, he told us about the genocide and how, in only twelve years, the people in Rwanda have come such a long way. They have developed their courts to bring people to justice, which may mean building a house or buying a cow and then allowing everyone to forgive each other and move forward. They are all Rwandans now. They have signs everywhere about the genocide so they will never forget and will continue to grow as a country. I was amazed by their strength to heal.

I had the privilege of visiting Rwanda to see the gorillas; it was another life-changing experience. Rwanda is a beautiful country with equally beautiful people, but its tragic history humbles you to the core. I will never forget sitting with a Tutsi guide in Kigali and listening to his firsthand accounts of the genocide. The resilience and strength of the people there are extraordinary.

The gorillas were fantastic. We were in the same area where Dian Fossey did her research, and there are ten habituated troops of gorillas, seven of which are used for tourism. Eight people hike up the mountain together once a day and can only stay for one hour. This minimizes the stress on the troop. We were only allowed an hour with the troop, and the time seemed to fly. The group we visited had been assigned to a different troop for research purposes, but when we found them, it was magic. Our troop's name was Amahora, which means "peace." There was a huge silverback, along with several babies and juvenile males. The silverback was named Ubumwa, which means "unity" in Rwanda. They were an easy troop to habituate. We were very close to the babies, and one juvenile male ran by and grabbed my leg in a playful yet powerful moment. His grip was strong, but his touch was so gentle as if he were aware of his strength, and he chose to be soft. Being so close to these incredible animals in their natural habitat was one of the most amazing moments of my life.

Seeing the gorillas on the most beautiful mountain, comfortable in their surroundings, brought tears to our eyes. They are true perfection and the picture of peace. Thankfully, their population has increased by fifteen percent in the last few years, so they are now up to seven hundred. I strongly recommend a trip to see them.

Next, we were off to Lewa in Kenya. I got to see all the people I knew there and all the animals, too. I massaged and rode the young horses I have known since they were born, and I did a follow-up massage class, too. I also saw Tula, a female black rhino, whom I worked on when she was six months old. She is too big for that now, but seeing her and her half-brother, whom I did get to scratch, was great. The sanctuary has really done a remarkable job of increasing the black rhino population.

In addition to these places, I've traveled to other parts of Africa many times. I've actually been to Tanzania more than Kenya, which still surprises me, considering how deeply my heart belongs to Kenya. My first trip to Tanzania was designed to be a very special one. I went there to see the chimpanzees, and I felt compelled to use the money my parents had left me for something unforgettable—something they would have wanted me to do. So, I set off on a once-in-a-lifetime adventure to Tanzania.

Ever since my trip to Rwanda, where I had seen the mountain gorillas, I dreamed of seeing chimpanzees. I find them fascinating on so many levels. My time as a zookeeper allowed me to study primate behavior, and my current role as an animal massage therapist drives me to evaluate muscle tone and structure on as many animals as possible.

The first few days were spent in a small, open-air hotel restaurant, eating alone and waiting for a plane to the preserve. Once there, I met an elderly couple who made the trip even more enjoyable. On our first day, we took a two-hour boat ride to the preserve. The Gombe Forest Stream is the most beautiful place I have seen. The lake is crystal clear; you can see all the way to the bottom. The water is pure and beautiful. It is representative of the wildlife that thrives on its shores.

After an hour and a half of climbing, we found our first chimpanzees. I was most impressed by the dominant male of this group, Ferdinand. His coat shone like black velvet, and his muscle structure was perfect. He was much larger than I expected and moved with power and grace. I watched his brother groom him, and their interactions were amazing, exciting, and very pleasant. Ferdinand quickly became one of my favorites.

During the next two days, we continued to see the chimpanzees. Ferdinand was a strong player in each day's visit. He became interested in his sister in a way that she was not interested in him, if you catch my drift. A female chimpanzee will not breed with her brother or her father, however. This did not make Ferdinand very happy. On the second day, Fanny and her baby, Fifty, climbed silently down a tree beside me. Ferdinand ran in front of me and went after her. They tussled in front of me for a few minutes, which gave me a great view of their muscles in action, not to mention some fabulous behavioral interaction.

Day three belongs to Fanny. That day's hike was short because the chimps were near the beach. Our first view was of a nervous male who stood cautiously watching us. My guide, Kapharr, kept us moving past him because our presence made him anxious. The consideration for their welfare was refreshing. Then they appeared! Fanny and her two young ones, along with a sub-adult male, made their way past us and stopped about eight feet away. Their interactions were beautiful and so loving as Fifty nursed and they groomed one another. It brings tears to your eyes to witness such a display of peace and contentment.

The chimpanzees were extraordinary. They're aggressive yet human-like in their behavior. While taking a picture of the pair, I felt a presence behind me. I turned to find a chimp walking just ten feet away, casually waving and continuing on its way. It was a surreal experience.

After visiting the chimpanzees for a few days, I went on a horseback-riding safari, which was truly life-changing. It was just me and the guides, and we had some of the most incredible wildlife encounters. The highlight was galloping alongside a giraffe, which was equally terrifying and exhilarating. My horse, a Russian pony, loved the chase and was determined to outrun the giraffe. I had no control, riding in a hackamore, but it didn't matter. At one point, I thought we might crash into a zebra or giraffe, but it was pure freedom.

We rode through valleys with animals surrounding us. When we stopped for a break, we looked up to see enormous herds of animals in the distance. Then, we galloped again, and thousands of animals started running alongside us. It was such a powerful feeling of unity with nature. The guides were so excited that they immediately called others when it was over to share in the experience.

I went back two more times after that and even became friends with the people who own Makao Farms. It's an experience I'll never forget—feeling free and connected to nature in a way I never thought possible.

I am so lucky to have gotten the chance to visit this piece of heaven on earth. I hope to return and bring others so they can see the beauty of life in Africa. The lessons I learned from these magnificent animals have and will continue to help me in my work at home.

Accepting Assistance

How I feel about living with vision loss really depends on the day. Some days are harder than others, and I can be pretty hard on myself for not trying to do more. I can't get a "normal" job so making money is challenging. I am grateful I am able to massage horses and dogs because I'm not able to do much else. As for my friends and family, everything feels pretty normal. No one treats me any differently, which is nice.

Sometimes I feel like my vision loss is a gift—like I can see the good things more clearly, and I can smell, hear, and feel so much more than other people. For example, when I was in Africa, I could hear animals all around me. I could hear them running, listen to their roars, and even hear them chewing. Other people couldn't hear that. I could smell animals while driving through the Serengeti—I could tell where an elephant was or hear a hawk somewhere. That was pretty cool.

Little things that most people never think twice about, like distinguishing between my toothbrush and my husband's, become daily challenges. I've used little tricks to help me, like putting rubber bands on the handles to tell them apart. And I've had to rely on others to help me navigate other simple things, like finding my seat on a plane or figuring out how to use public transportation or apps like Uber. It's frustrating, especially since I wasn't raised in the age of technology. I didn't grow up learning how to use smartphones and apps. Now the world is full of tech, and it feels like I'm always behind. I enjoy many things, but reading, writing, or using the computer more easily would be awesome.

Driving is one of the biggest challenges. I can't drive, and I'll never be able to. So it's hard to meet friends because you can't drive them somewhere or pick anything up for them. I feel like I can't offer much other than myself. I've considered the existing driving programs, but my vision is too poor for them to be safe or possible. It's hard not to be able to go where I want, when I want, without relying on others. Things as simple as going to a restaurant and trying to read the menu are challenging. When I'm alone, stopping somewhere to grab food is difficult because I can't see what I'm ordering. Once, at an airport, I had to deal with a self-checkout kiosk, and I just couldn't do it. I couldn't see what I was supposed to select. Sometimes, even simple things like adjusting the thermostat are a struggle. I can't tell the temperature without taking a picture to ensure I'm setting it correctly.

Even with these challenges, I am able to stay incredibly active. Playing catch is tough because I'll see the ball coming, and then lose track of it completely. It's frustrating when the ball hits me in the face, but I've learned to laugh at myself through those moments. I like to walk the dogs and ride horses. With the dogs, I can still run agility with no issue. I know the course, walk it, and feel its flow. The dogs and I are a team. They've become my eyes in many ways. I can't always see the course map or sometimes the numbers on the course, so I have to follow someone around. But once I do the course, I'm fine—my version of "fine," anyway. With jumping horses, it's a little more complicated. I've learned to walk the ring and map out the jumps in my mind, but I still sometimes miss a fence, especially since I have a blind spot in the center of my vision. I rely on landmarks for jumping and agility—large trees, the corners of buildings, poles, or other prominent structures. These are my guides, and they help me navigate the course so I can line up with the jumps properly. I'm constantly adapting and finding new ways to make things work.

My vision is progressively declining due to the disease, and every day I notice small changes. My mother started me early on with strategies to hopefully prevent it from getting as bad as it could. There are things I've done for years that I'm still able to do, but it's becoming more apparent that my vision is getting worse. For example, I used to think I was giving someone a twenty dollar bill, only to realize I had handed them a fifty dollar bill. Moments like these remind me of the challenges I face, so I've had to limit certain things I do to keep from making mistakes. But my vision is still expected to continue to deteriorate until it's completely gone. So I try to go to as many places as possible and do as many things as possible to make the most of my time. Even with my vision limitations, I keep pushing forward, learning to adjust, and continuing to do the things that bring me joy—riding, training, and competing. It's not easy, but I wouldn't have it any other way. People take so many things for granted, and I feel that weight every day.

Beyond the everyday challenges, it's incredibly frustrating when I can't see things like minor cuts or scratches on my animals like I used to. I've always been so attuned to their needs. I rely on my sense of smell—if there's a cut, even as small as a scratch, I can often smell it. It's an odd ability, but it works. Still, being unable to check things with certainty without any assistance—like having to take a picture on my phone or ask my husband—like I used to, is one of the hardest aspects. My goal now is to get to a point where I can hire someone to help me care for the animals properly if I completely lose my vision; someone who can make sure I'm not missing anything important.

The little things—the things most people never have to think about—weigh on me. But in my heart, I know I can still make the most of every moment, every experience, and every day. My goal is to travel, see the world, and experience as much as I can before my sight fades completely. I may not be able to see the birds, animals, or smiles as clearly, but I have the gift of imagination and memories. I'm holding on to those.

Part Two
The Accident

Siri Saved Me

I had a terrible accident on July 25, 2023. That morning, I rode three horses. I spent about ten minutes walking and trotting on Cake, then rode my paint horse, Penzi, who is such a good girl. I had a little bit of time left to ride Sugar, a fourteen-year-old chestnut Oldenburg mare who came to me about two years prior. When I got her, she had only received basic training and had lost her sparkle. However, with time and care, she had turned into a beautiful jumper and was fun to ride.

I was riding Sugar in my arena, and I was in a hurry. The day was very busy for me, and I only had fifteen minutes to ride, so it was a short, conditioning ride. That day, my two-year-old fillies were around, and when one of them ran to the fence, it distracted Sugar. As I rode her down the arena, I felt that something wasn't quite right. I wondered what was going on. I kept cantering around the first corner, but as I reached the next corner, Sugar suddenly fell onto her side, right on top of me.

At first, I wasn't sure if we both fell; that's how fast it happened. I never felt like I was falling; the whole experience was something I had never encountered before. It all happened so quickly, like getting rear-ended or punched in the face when you don't see it coming. I'd fallen off horses many times since I started riding when I was two, but never like this.

I hit the ground so hard that my ear was ringing, and I couldn't hear anything. It was like a bomb had gone off. Everything went black and I couldn't move. The weird thing was I couldn't understand why I couldn't move. I felt like I was still on Sugar, but I didn't understand why that would be. I figured it was bad and that I couldn't move because I had probably broken my neck. I tried not to freak out, which wasn't that hard because I didn't have a lot of options. All I knew was that I couldn't move, see, or scream. I thought, *Don't move, whatever you do, don't move.* I remembered what my mom told me back when I had broken my back: "When you break your back, don't move a muscle." So, I didn't.

Then I remember thinking it'd be OK because the guy coming to spray the weeds in the pasture and the arena would see me, and everything would be fine. So I just lay there and tried not to move. I don't know if I fell asleep or passed out. Literally a second before the accident, I had looked at my phone and saw it was around 10:15 a.m.

The next thing I knew, I was on my back instead of my right side, and I was roasting in the sun. I could hear Sugar grazing beside me, and I wanted to look at her, but then I remembered not to move a muscle. It turned out to be almost an hour later. I knew this because my phone beeped when I got a text message about getting a haircut. That made me realize I could try using Siri to call for help. "Hey, Siri," I said, "call 911." Thankfully, it worked. Speaking very softly with shallow breathing, I managed to get out the address, what happened, and approximately where I was. Almost immediately after that, I found myself unable to breathe. I remember saying to the 911 operator that I was dying and that I couldn't breathe.

Just Breathe

My friends Walker and Melinda heard the call because Walker is a volunteer first responder, and he immediately sent Melinda over to my house. Meanwhile, I was still on the phone with the 911 operator, unable to move. I was having a lot of trouble breathing and couldn't take a deep breath, which made it difficult to swallow.

When Melinda arrived, she told me it took her a few minutes to find me. She came and sat by me, and I kept thinking, *Why is she not brushing the sand off my face? Why is she not covering my face? I'm burning up in the sand and the sun.* But she just sat by me. She took my phone out of my pants pocket and called Ken, my husband. "You've got to get here!" she told him. "It's bad; it's really bad."

I remember saying to her, "I'm gonna die. I can't breathe." I wanted to tell her to tell Ken that I loved him and that I couldn't imagine my life without him, but I didn't. I could practically hear my mom saying, "Maria, stop being so dramatic. You're not dying; you're just injured. You're not dying, so just stop it."

Later, Melinda told me that when she first found me, I looked like a pile of rags, and it was obvious that my neck was broken. Thankfully, she knew not to touch or move me.

As I lay there baking in the sun, I suffered what I thought were burns on my legs from my riding pants. All I could think about was my husband and what I wanted to say to him. But I couldn't bring myself to say it, because I didn't want to give up. I remember consciously telling myself to breathe, forcing myself to take the deepest breaths I could muster.

For some reason, I also remembered that time when my brother Kevin said to me, "You can see now. You're just not trying." It made me want to try harder. So, I sat there, not moving a muscle, and mentally focusing on breathing, just in and out.

Just breathe. That's when everything went blank. At that point, I was no longer breathing and had no pulse.

Melinda and our neighbor Jim held onto Sugar, who stood close to me the entire time I was down. They didn't want her to get spooked and cause any more damage or hurt herself, so they put her away. I'm sure they believed I would be dead by the time the firefighters arrived.

Don't Move

Two firefighters and one volunteer responded to the call. Walker called for a second ambulance, and it was actually the second one that arrived first on the scene. If he had not done that, the ambulance would have been too late, and I would not have survived. When they found me, I was blue, my pulse oximeter reading was 81, I had no pulse, and I wasn't breathing. The only way they could resuscitate me was through straight oxygen. If they had tried to do any CPR due to my neck fracture, I would have been dead. Thank God they knew that.

A few days later, they told me that I only had a few minutes left before it would be too late. As gross as it is, Melinda told me my neck was obviously broken, which probably saved my life as well. If they hadn't seen that I had a broken neck, they might've moved me. If my mother hadn't taught me not to move when I get injured, I'd be dead. If I had looked at my horse, I'd be dead. My bones would've jammed into my brain and killed me. If there was ever a day when everything went right when everything had gone wrong, that was it.

While I was passed out, they were able to slide a neck collar underneath me to stabilize my neck. As Jim and Melinda stood there watching, my husband, Ken, was still on the phone, and he wanted to know what was going on. Ken had been driving, so he pulled the car over. He asked if I was still alive, and Jim was silent. Thankfully, the responders got me breathing again. They told me I screamed when I woke up. When Jim heard me scream, he told Ken I was still alive, so he pulled back out on the road to meet me at the hospital. The joke was that, clearly, I was on my way to hell, and that's why I was screaming. Other people would probably say, well, she never shuts her mouth, so that's why she was screaming. I'm fairly certain I was screaming when I woke up because I was trying so hard to breathe.

They had to carry me to the ambulance because they couldn't get it into my pasture where I was down. When I first woke up, I was speaking gibberish. But when they were loading me into the ambulance, I could speak more clearly. All I remember about being in the ambulance was talking to Loretta, and that I was happy that I could move my arms and legs again. One of the paramedics said, "Hey, how about you don't move so much?" The next thing I remember is being in the emergency room.

They took me to the level-one trauma unit. I don't remember my first CT scan or first MRI. I just remember a nurse coming in and saying, "Do you know this handsome gentleman?" Just then, my husband walked through the door. As he walked down the hall, I laughed and said, "I've never seen him before in my life." I can't imagine what it was like for him that day.

Actually, I can because nearly a year to the day, I saved his life in a pool when he had a seizure. It was terrifying. I thought he was going to die. If I had slipped, if I hadn't thought to hold him up, he would've drowned. My life has been hard since we moved to Aiken. I guess it's what was supposed to happen, and it could've been a lot harder for both of us.

Two or three doctors came in shortly after my husband arrived. At first, they said they had good news, and that I'd just have to have a brace on for six months. I thought, *Sweet, I can do that.* They thought they could just put a brace on to stabilize my neck. But soon they realized that the bones were moving and that I would need surgery the next day. Apparently, I had shattered my C2, the same fracture that Christopher Reeve had.

From there, I went for a CT scan. I cannot begin to tell you the amount of pain I felt when they had to move me for the scan and then eventually for the MRI that evening. It was excruciating, and the medical staff had to work so hard to make sure I didn't move. When I broke my back when I was ten (L1), I had to remain perfectly still for two weeks, but that was nothing compared to this. If I had moved the wrong way, something could have gone wrong, and I could have been killed by bones pressing into my brain. I didn't know all that then, but I knew it was bad.

They held up a board with a paper for me to sign to consent to surgery. Basically, it said the risks of my surgery were death and paralysis. I signed it, of course. What are you going to do? It's not like I could walk out and find another doctor. I don't think Ken realized what I was saying to him at that moment, but I told him I could not survive if I were paralyzed. I can't be blind and paralyzed. It's just too much. A lot of my freedom is based on motion. I didn't know what I would do. I can't say that I was thinking positively or negatively; I wasn't even scared. It was like, for once in my life, what was going to happen would happen. I had done all I could at that point.

Ken stayed with me until late in the evening, but we had horses and dogs to care for, and he needed to get some sleep. We talked about nothing and everything—what to do with the animals, how much we loved each other, etc. He wanted to come back in the morning for surgery, but it's a forty-five-minute drive, one way. It was also a five- to six-hour surgery, and the operation was scheduled for seven a.m. I figured it would be better if he didn't worry about driving so early and just stayed home with the dogs.

I didn't sleep much that night, if at all. I couldn't have eaten if I wanted to, but I didn't want to. They had to do another MRI, and I can't tell you how excruciatingly painful it was when they moved me. I've never felt pain like that. I screamed and cried. I was terrified when they had to move me. It was just horrible. If I had known how dangerous it was, I would've been even more frightened. "Don't move," the nurses told me. "Don't help us. We'll do everything." So, I didn't move a muscle. Anyone who knows me knows that letting go of control is not my forte, but in a life-or-death situation, you do what you need to do.

In the morning, I dictated a will—what to do with the animals and where they should go if something happened to me, as well as how much I love Ken and what I thought he should do. God knows how coherent it was. I always thought that if anything like that ever happened to me, where I was dying, I would think about my animals, about riding and playing with the dogs. But I didn't. I just thought about Ken.

Stop Being Dramatic

The doctors came in around five, and then the anesthesiologist came in. At first, they just stood there and looked at me. Then they looked at each other, whispered to each other, and then continued looking at me. Meanwhile, I was lying there thinking the surgery would be like when I had my elbow operated on after falling out of a hayloft. When I had that surgery, the surgical team joked and laughed with me and said, "Mexican Irish? We gotta load you up." These guys, however, weren't joking. There was nothing funny about what they were about to tell me. Inching up to the side of the bed, they told me they were going to have to intubate me while I was awake, because if they put me under, it would kill me. Without skipping a beat, I looked up at them and said, "Well, awake sounds like a great idea then." Then they just wheeled me off.

I remember getting wheeled to the operating room. All the other times I've been operated on, I've been terrified. Not this time. I didn't even take in much of it. I don't know if it was the pain or what. I guess that's just what happens when you decide to let go.

Lots of doctors were waiting for me in the operating room. I don't know how many, maybe five or six, along with two or three anesthesiologists. When they put that tube down my throat, it was unbearable. I have a really strong gag reflex, and I remember thinking, *Do not move, Maria. You're going to die. Just let it happen. Just do it. Don't get upset. Don't get sick. Just suck it up. Like Mom always said, "Stop being dramatic."* It's strange to credit your survival to a woman who's been gone for years. I don't have any way to tell her that what she taught me saved my life, but I think she knows.

I woke up in the ICU with Ken right beside me. Thankfully, I was not a bit sick, which was good because I certainly didn't want to be throwing up. They let me get up almost immediately.

Obviously, I was super weak and terrified to do anything wrong. I didn't want to fall. I wasn't allowed to turn my head, not that I could. The collar was very uncomfortable and dug into the back of my head. They ended up changing the collar because it was too big, and the padding was inadequate. I was still plastered with sand from being in the arena. It was buried in my hair and all over me. There were also these large blisters on my leg, and nobody could figure out how they got there or what they were. To say I was miserable would be an understatement.

That said, I felt so much better. My neck didn't even hurt when they moved me to do the other CT scan after the surgery. Overall, the care I received in the ICU was incredible—second to none. I will never forget the staff's kindness, compassion, and attention to detail, and I will forever be grateful for their dedication to others. The nurses were amazing. They brushed my hair and washed off what they could. They simply were caring, good people. I wanted for nothing when I was in the ICU, but sadly, that ended around 10 p.m. after the surgery, and they moved me in with the general population.

If the ICU was a five-star hotel, the regular floor was a living nightmare. It was an old hospital, and it was dreadful. I never saw my roommate, but apparently, she was chained to the bed and often screamed that she was being raped, which was clearly untrue. She was absolutely awful. I felt bad for her in a way, to be that upset and confused. My nurse was terrible, too. She helped me walk to the bathroom, where I proceeded to throw up my pain pills. Of course, I couldn't bend over, so I told her I needed to throw them up in a pan or something. She just looked at me, disgusted, hoping that I didn't get anything on her. I was just afraid that I was going to move my neck the wrong way and kill myself. After that, I didn't get any pain pills, I didn't get any food, I didn't get a drink—nothing. I just lay there in my bed, where I couldn't sleep because I was so uncomfortable, so miserable, and had to listen to the woman next to me scream.

What I remember most about being on the regular floor was how everyone who came in looked at me strangely. The rehab people came in and tried to give me some exercises for my right arm, which was definitely weak. I couldn't even use a fork. My leg seemed OK, besides the giant blisters on my right thigh. When the folks from neurosurgery came in, I remember my doctor looking at me and again saying, "You have Christopher Reeve's fracture. You are very lucky. You'll be seeing me a lot." I just smiled and said, "OK." He then told me that I'd be able to ride in nine months, which I was thrilled to hear at the time, because I thought he would say I would never ride again.

The next day, Thursday, July 27th, I was released from the hospital. It was amazing. I had undergone major neck surgery, yet my hospital stay was just two days. That said, I was petrified to leave. I could walk, but not with any kind of confidence. I remained frightened the entire drive home.

265 Days Until I Can Ride

The drive home itself was a nightmare. Any bump we hit hurt and scared me. I was terrified of getting into a car accident. Riding in the car was terrifying, getting in and out of the car was terrifying, and walking into the house was terrifying. Every single thing I did felt scary because I kept thinking that if I made one wrong move, I could die. I tried to feed myself after not eating on Tuesday or Wednesday, and it felt like I'd had a stroke because I couldn't use my right arm. Even ten or eleven days later, I still had some weakness in that arm and hand.

Being home was an adventure. I decreased my medication because I felt sick and out of it the whole time. I couldn't sleep at night. The sores on my leg were killing me, and it hurt so bad to lie down. It felt like my leg was going to split open. So, I paced around all night, crying half the time as I tried to get comfortable. I dreaded nighttime and looked forward so much to seeing the sun come up because it meant I could get up. It was awful.

That said, I hate complaining because I'm not complaining—I'm alive, and there's nothing I can even begin to say about that.

Journal Entry 8/7/2023

I feel better today. I was unable to sleep and cried most of the night, but I feel better now. I feel stronger; my legs feel stronger and better on my feet. I'm worried I did something wrong to my neck because I had to lie on my side for a while, which I'm not supposed to do without a pillow. Ken wasn't there to tell me if my neck was straight. I don't sit still enough for him to sleep in the bedroom at night. It's too much up and down, and I have to sleep sitting up on the bed now. But so far, today is a better day, and I'm walking faster. Heading over to see Dylan now. I love looking at my horses in the field. It sucks that starting next week, two of them will head off to their temporary homes.

A couple of days after I got home, the firefighters came to see me. They looked at me like I was a ghost. I can't imagine what it was like for them to see someone who was that blue and foaming at the mouth. It must be so stressful trying to determine if someone is going to live or die. I hope they understood how much their actions that day positively affected me, my animals, my friends, and my family. The fact that they take time out of their lives to help others is the most amazing thing ever, and I am so grateful to them every day.

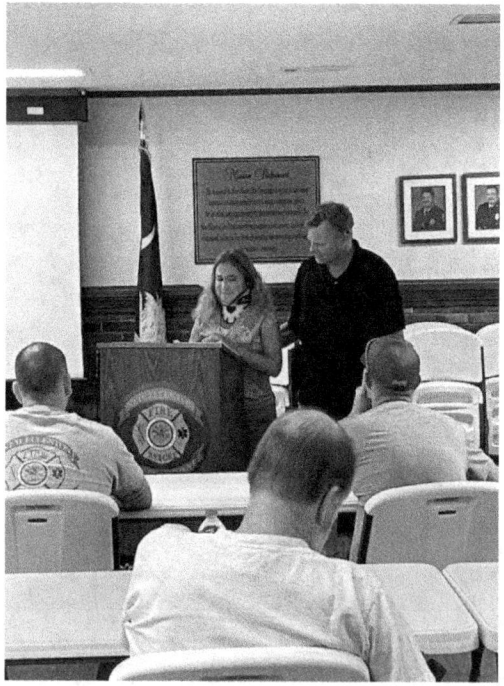

Facebook Post 8/9/2023
Ken and I went last night to thank the New Ellenton Fire Department for saving my life on July 25. It is a small department made up of mostly volunteers. I wanted to thank them for giving their time to help others in the community. I really wanted to let them know how important their sacrifice is.

After I got home, I went back and forth from wanting to recover to feeling frustrated, because I couldn't ride or run with my dogs in agility. Then I thought about how grateful I was to be alive, and I reminded myself that I had been minutes away from not being here anymore. I still wonder why I survived. What am I supposed to do now with my life? I feel that I'm meant to do something magical; I'm just not sure what. I hear stories of others not making it, and I don't understand why I'm here and they're not.

This was not how I pictured this year to go. Now I'm in a desperate search for purpose. Everyone keeps telling me to open up to what's coming, but it's hard. As I write this, I still have 265 more days until I can ride my horse.

Part Three
Recovery

Hardest Thing Ever

I don't talk much about my rehab because I never recognized all the small steps until they became bigger. It was important to me to maintain my physical well-being, so when I first came home and was using a walker to inch a few feet at a time, I used a gift card that a good friend had given me to order bicycle pedals. That may sound strange, but they were to be used while sitting in a chair so you can pedal anywhere. I couldn't lift any weight at all, so that was out of the question. The doctor told me that if I hadn't been so physically fit before the accident, I probably would have died. So, I knew it was important to stay in shape. I also knew I would be looking at three hard weeks of recovery for each week of downtime if I didn't at least do some light movement.

Once the doctor removed the staples from my hip and neck in early August, I was allowed to walk as much as I could tolerate. Unfortunately, that was not very much in the beginning. I couldn't walk my dogs on leashes, so I had to walk alone most of the time. Occasionally, my neighbors would join me, which was wonderful. I was very slow and unsteady at first, but it worked. I started walking just a few feet outside holding onto the fence. I walked a little further each time, with a stick for support, because I could not risk falling. After some time, I was finally able to walk to the end of my street and back. I didn't even notice the improvement until I looked back at how I'd started. I remember the day I made it to the corner. Some neighbors were riding by on their horses, and they said, "Maria, is that you?" I must've looked atrocious.

I still couldn't go too far, though, because I got tired and didn't want to push it. I couldn't twist, bend down, move my head at all, or lift anything. My number two cervical vertebrae had been broken into several pieces (at least five, I think), and the doctor said that it was a challenge to pin them together. They had to take a piece of my hip bone to fuse vertebra one and two, and used screws to connect the other pieces of the vertebra. Some pieces still aren't completely fused, but my doctor is hopeful that as the bone heals, they will come together. In his opinion, the only way that such trauma could've happened was if something major occurred, like Sugar stepping on me when she got up, or her rolling on me in the process of getting up. Since it was only that vertebrae, I continued to mend.

Those days at home following the accident were the hardest I've ever had. I couldn't do anything that made me who I was. My head hurt if I did too much, and I was scared that if I pushed myself too far, I'd never be able to walk, move my arms, ride, or be myself again. It was terrifying to be so vulnerable. I'd worked so hard my whole life not to depend on others. My whole life had been a struggle for independence and survival, and now I was in the biggest struggle I'd ever faced, both mentally and physically.

When in-home physical therapy came, I was excited. I thought they would give me a lot of things to do like weights and stretching, but instead, they gave me a Tupperware container full of rice. I couldn't feel anything with my fingers, so I had to sift through that with my hands to find the plastic pieces of different shapes and sizes that were hidden in the rice. This was supposed to help with my dexterity, especially in my right hand. Physical therapy rehab for my right hand and arm also involved sifting through sand to find marbles and blocks, squeezing Styrofoam blocks, playing with putty, and stacking cups. My right arm was too weak even to lift it, so I did exercises where I'd walk my right arm up the wall to make it stronger. Being a massage therapist and not having feeling or dexterity in my hands was surreal. So I worked very hard on that exercise and squeezed the therapeutic putty to strengthen my hands. With each passing day, I felt a little bit stronger. Of course, I had both good and bad days, and the whole experience was a lot to take in.

A month after the accident, I could finally put my hair in a ponytail by myself. It was a huge victory on the slow but steady climb back to my normal physical condition. We celebrated a big milestone when I was able to put my hair up by myself. Both Ken and I were grateful that I could finally do my own ponytails. It was definitely a victory to celebrate! All of the tools I used to regain what I lost were not only valuable physically but also mentally, because they gave me a goal to shoot for and something to do during the day.

For nine months, I wasn't allowed to lift anything, so everything I did had to be lightweight. After a while, I started a daily regimen of squats using one-pound weights on a limited basis. Sometimes, I would just practice moving my arms.

I enjoyed exercising to Tom Petty songs because many of them resonated with me. The first one I really connected with was "Angel Dream." I loved the line where he says, "Cut my lifeline when drifting through space." Ken would play the guitar part for this song, and I would sing along. It gave me something to do. Singing was difficult since I couldn't move my head, but the song made me feel good, like I wasn't alone. As I was able to do more and more on my personalized workout program, I would listen to "I Won't Back Down" and work out with one-pound weights. I'd squat and turn around in a small space with something to grab in case I lost my balance. This became my theme song. I posted a video on Instagram of me wearing my neck brace while doing my workout, and I also played it on my first real day of riding Sugar as a musical freestyle. The music was great; the freestyle part, though, was not so good.

After coming home, my favorite parts of the day were when I was doing virtual massages or in-person evaluations. It was so helpful for me to feel like I could still make a difference. I spent most of my days walking. When I felt up to it, I tried to walk for at least an hour a day and brush my quieter horses.

The severity of my cervical break made rehab slow and difficult. I needed to take time to heal. That said, anyone who knows me knows patience is not my virtue, so I tried to push myself as hard as I could without going over the edge. The pain caused by the pressure sores on my leg from when the horse was lying on top of me made it difficult to do normal things. I couldn't even sleep because of the pain. It was so bad that, for a long time, I could only wear skirts. It felt like my leg was going to split in half.

For probably two months, nobody knew what the blister-like marks were, so they went untreated until I went to wound care. Thankfully, they got me on the right track. Before I got help, however, the sores were insanely painful, making moving or even sitting very difficult. This was probably a good thing, though, because I was unable to push myself too hard. Today, I still feel like I am not one hundred percent. Once the sores and my balance improved, though, I began to get my confidence back.

I was beginning to sleep a little bit better, and the pressure sore on my right leg was healing. Every day was an improvement, as I continued my countdown—262 days until I could ride.

This was the hardest thing I'd ever been through, and I kept looking at what was on the other side. I wanted to get there so badly, so I just kept trying, hoping I was doing the right things. Simple things like sleeping, getting up, and brushing my teeth were hard. Life had always been hard for me with my vision issues, but this was a whole new level of hard. All the support that I got along the way made it possible for me to keep going.

I just wanted to be me again. I guess that's what drove me; it's always driven me. What made this experience so hard was that everything that was easy for me before, everything that had gotten me through life up to that point, was hard or simply not possible now, and that was terrifying. My sense of balance and awareness had always been my saving grace, and now I didn't have it. Or at the very least, I had to build it back up.

I may have given the illusion to some that what I was going through was easy, but it was not. I'd been in some pretty tough spots before, but nothing like this. If it wasn't for my insane drive to get back to riding my horses and running my dogs in agility, I don't know if I would have had the drive to do anything other than sit in my room in the dark.

Some days were more challenging than others. It wasn't so much the pain in my stupid leg or that damn pressure sore, it was the constant discomfort and fear of making a mistake. Sometimes I had a hard time just getting up. Just trying to be more normal was frightening. I felt vulnerable, and I knew if I got knocked down or pushed, I'd be in trouble. If I got in a car accident, I'd also be in trouble.

I spent entire days working out, walking, and doing whatever little weights I could to stay strong and be more normal. I knew this time wouldn't last forever, but sometimes it felt like it would. I knew I shouldn't be complaining because I was alive. But you know what? Sometimes I needed the right to complain. I literally counted the minutes until my next doctor's appointment. I needed a good report. I just needed something to change, something to improve in any way.

Facebook Post 9/6/2023
Well, time for an update. Just leaving the doctor's office; x-ray looks good. I can take the brace off when I'm sitting in the house. I can try to sleep without it. I'm allowed to use a pillow—that's exciting! I still can only lift as much as a gallon of milk. Nothing else is really changed, but at least everything's on the right track. He thought I was insane when I asked him about running, lol. He's gonna talk to me about that when I see him in six weeks.

Facebook Post 9/27/2023
Week nine update—not too much exciting news to report; just waiting until October 19, which is my next appointment. I am getting bored with my crate rest, lol. This is kind of the hardest part. I feel good, not 100%, but I still am not allowed to lift anything or twist or turn or bend, so it's a little frustrating. The best news is that the pressure sores on my leg are finally healing, so the constant pain I had in my leg is beginning to go away. That means I can sleep, which will make Ken very happy. I'll be a little less testy.

I spend my days walking, sometimes up to 22,000 steps a day. I've also begun to ride a recumbent bike in the clubhouse, just trying to stay fit. I'm doing basic exercises still with my right arm, like just getting to lift over my head and out to the side. It's improved, but still slightly weak. I have slight numbness still in a few of my fingers. The feeling in the back of my head seems like it's slowly coming back, and also in my hips, so hopefully, that will be the case. I have also begun working on the psychological aspect of going through a trauma like this, which is good because that will also only help with my healing process. Thank you again, everybody, for all your support.

No Backing Down

After the accident, all I could think about was getting back to my horses. It was about a week before I could enter the barn area. My house is a hunt box style, so my barn is attached to the house. It's not like I had to walk far, but being on the walker and very unsteady, I was unable to get out there until a week after the accident. When I did, all I could do was pet them. They had to be in the cross-ties, so the only horse I trusted was Chocolate Cake. I couldn't have any of them hit me in the head or move their feet too quickly and knock me down. My husband put Chocolate Cake in the cross-ties so I could pet her.

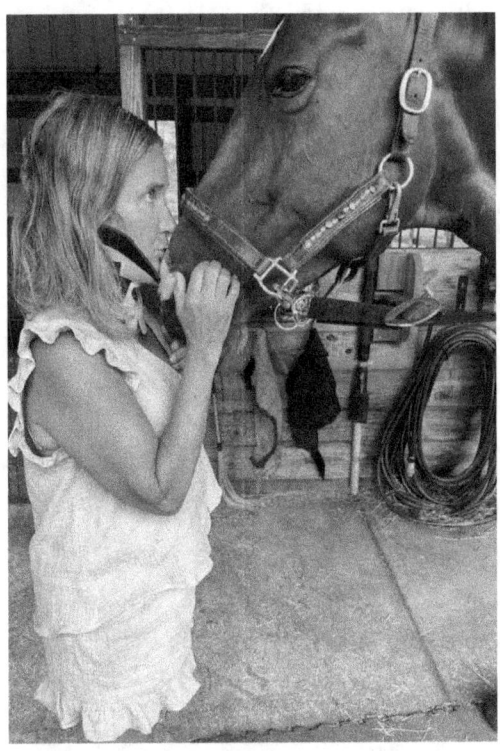

Facebook Post 7/30/2023
Thanks for all the support, it truly made a difference.
I always knew Chocolate Cake was the best medicine.

That was my first go with the horses. From then on, I was able to feed them and do other things. I had to lease two of my horses after the accident, which was so hard for me, but we didn't have any money because I couldn't work, and they needed to be spoiled and loved. As the days passed, I started to get the itch to ride. I was not cleared to do so, however, until January or February. It was supposed to be nine months before I could ride again, but I missed it so much. I missed the feel; I missed everything about it. Because of my eye situation, riding gives me freedom. I can see when I'm riding because the horses can see what I can't.

I missed the feeling and comfort of being on a horse so much that I made my husband bring this giant stuffed horse, which was designed for kids to sit on, and put it in my living room. Then, I could at least sit on something that felt like a horse.

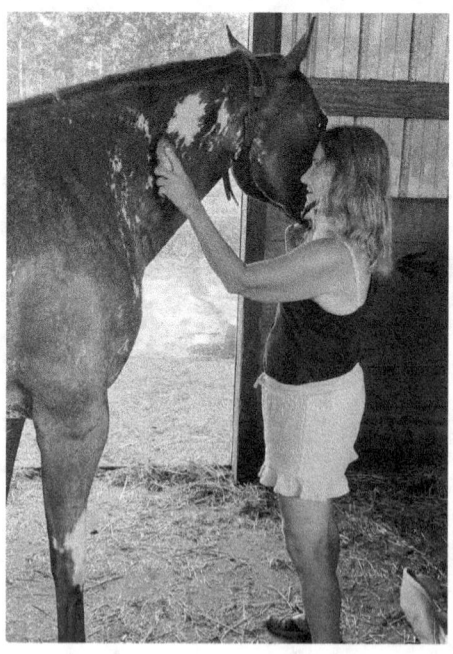

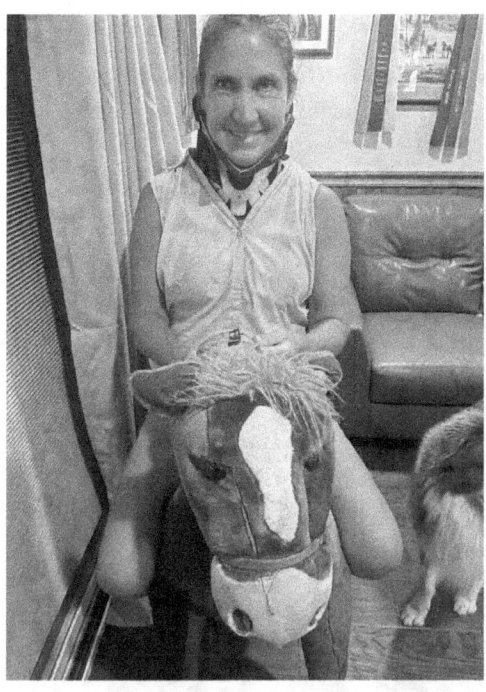

From there, I had my barn help—the person who helped me with stalls—hold my old horse so I could just sit on him. Dylan, who is thirty-five, is short and rock solid. I would get on and off with the help of a tall mounting block. From there, I would put him in the cross-ties. As I could start doing more with the horses, I would drag a chair over, climb on him, and sit on his back with him in the cross-ties. I couldn't get jerked or pulled at all, and I had no strength, so I couldn't do anything more than that.

One day, my husband left the house and saw me sitting on Dylan's back with him cross-tied in the aisle. He just shook his head and kept walking. When I asked him if it made him nervous that I would ride again, he said he always knew I would. In the very beginning, I knew I would too.

Facebook Post 8/24/2023

Sugar says hello. My friend who got here first the day of my accident said she stood right beside me, just dripping with sweat. Such a good horse.

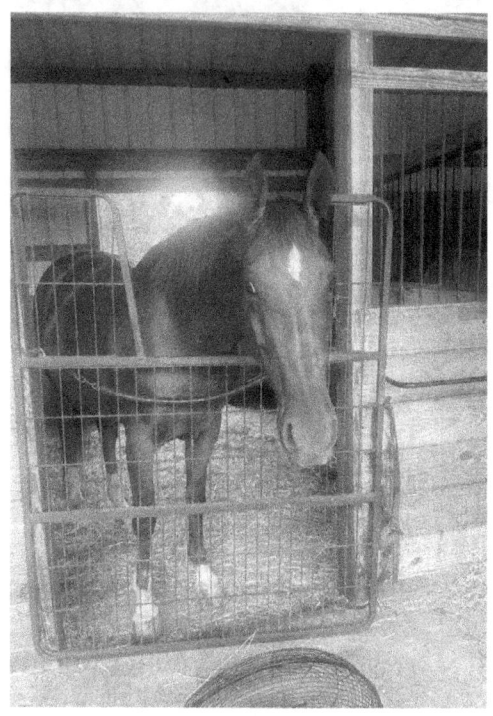

Facebook Post 10/19/2023

Well, the much-awaited doctor's appointment is over, and everything looks great. He said it's healed straight, and I can start lifting as much as I want as long as I don't strain myself, like I can't feel any pulling on my neck. I can leave the collar off unless I'm in a position where I might fall, which, since I'm around horses and dogs a lot, is kind of a lot, lol. I'm allowed to start running! I can do agility. I have exercises to do to get my neck to turn, which is very strange. He is going to do a CAT scan on January 18, and the results of that CAT scan will let me know if I can ride earlier or not. He's only doing a CAT scan since I am so active. He wants to make sure that everything is in good condition, which is the best-case scenario from today's appointment.

When I was allowed to take off the neck brace except when driving or walking, I decided that meant I could ride. The doctor said I could run, so I figured, what's the difference? I tried jogging, but that didn't go so well. Riding was a different story. I mostly walked and did a little trotting and cantering. What I noticed most was that my whole body would shake if they hit a divot or something in the ground. I had no core strength or upper body strength. I still wasn't allowed to lift anything over ten pounds. I just didn't have the strength and stamina to actually ride.

The climb back to riding wasn't as easy as I thought. I wanted to get on, and I loved to ride, so I was excited to do it. But I would often feel a total sense of terror. It was especially bad when I was cantering, and I would picture being in total darkness and unable to move, which was my first memory of the accident. If I felt like a foot wasn't going to be placed correctly, I would panic a little bit. This fear has faded, but it hasn't completely gone away. There are days and moments when it is still very fresh in my mind. I need to continue with some therapy to get past that emotional trauma, but I continue to push through it on my own as well.

Facebook Post 10/29/23
I'm being safe with my brace on, and I rode the merry-go-round at the fair. It felt awesome, LOL!

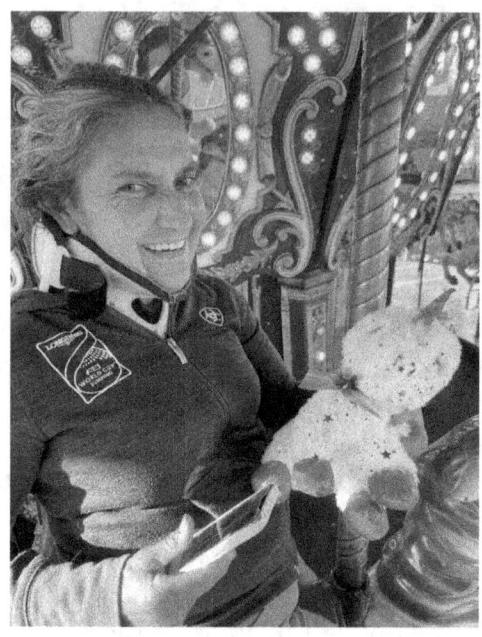

My first debut ride was at Good Fortune Farms for their Festivus party. I rode Sugar, the horse that fell on me, in the "Save the Champagne" ride. I did a musical dressage test to Tom Petty's "I Won't Back Down," which became my theme during my recovery. It was the song I first began dancing to in the house and while working out as I tried to get stronger. It was the perfect song for my first ride back. I was crying during the entire ride because it felt so good. I also took Sugar over some cross rails in the jumper jackpot class that day. The classes were just for fun, but I was the winner because I was so happy on my horse. It felt so good. Finally, I had some normalcy.

Facebook Post 11/19/2023
First, I'm back. I got to do a musical freestyle at Good Fortune Farms. It was amazing to be back on her, by the way. Now I'll call her the crusher, lol. Sugar was great, and it felt really good to ride again. Thanks, everyone, again, for all your support. It means the world to me. Without you guys, I would not be where I am today. Thank you.

Facebook Post 11/20/2023
One more picture from the awesome day at Good Fortune Farms yesterday, the don't spill the champagne ride. Sugar did not care for champagne spilling on her. I'm not sure if you can tell, but I'm super happy I'm riding.

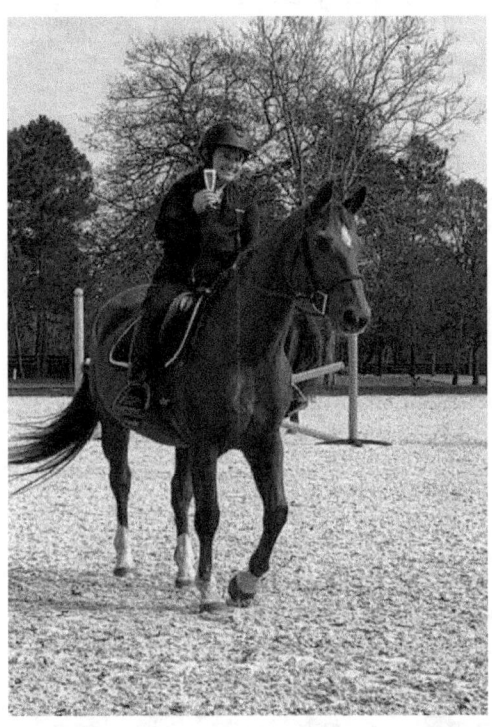

For some reason, starting back to real jumping made me nervous, even though our fall didn't happen while jumping. I knew I couldn't let myself fall at that point. I wore a safety vest in case I did, but I also had to ride defensively.

My first show in the spring was so much fun. I didn't do very well, but it was something I had to do. I wasn't ready, but I had to push myself to do it mentally, and it made me feel good. Jumping on my horses is one of my favorite things, and I hope I always can. I think another reason I felt so pushed and driven was because I didn't know when I might wake up and not be able to see at all. Hopefully, that day will never come, but I must live like it might, as I continue to push myself and keep trying.

Overcoming this accident has made me believe that if the worst does happen with my eyesight, I will be able to push past it and succeed. Now I'm back to jumping and riding my horses, and I have even backed my filly. I'm still not one hundred percent in terms of riding confidence, and I don't know if I ever will be, but I keep trying every day because I love it.

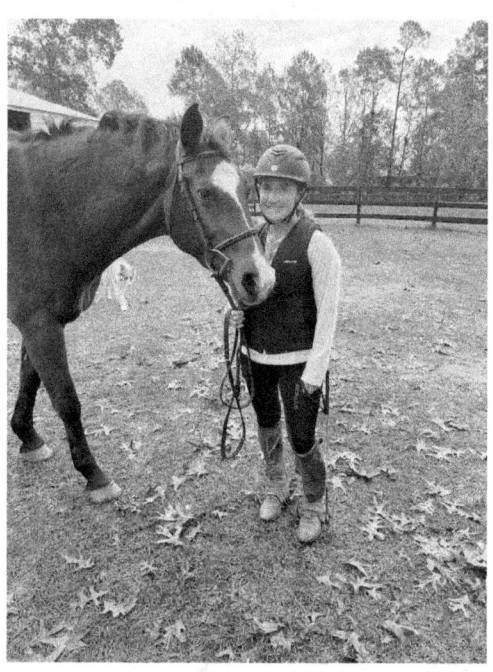

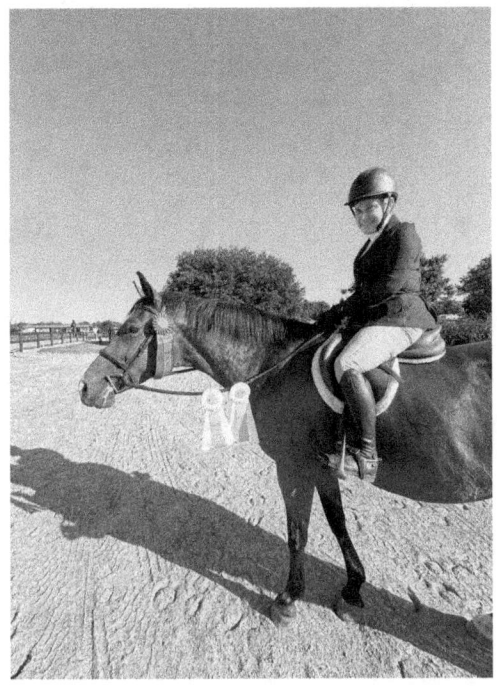

Time Heals

I could not even be with my dogs much my first night home. When they first saw me after the accident, they growled. I guess they feared me because they didn't know what had happened to me. I had to use a walker to get into my house. It wasn't very far, but my husband had to help me. I could not allow myself to get knocked over by a dog, so we had them separated. That first day, they were behind an X-pen outside my bedroom door, and I slowly introduced myself to them one at a time. Slide, my red merle, was first, and then I just kind of went down the list from there.

I wasn't afraid of my dogs, but they are rambunctious, fun, and driven, and they're used to a lot of activity and exercise. So, I was worried they would knock me down. I couldn't bend over, and I couldn't look up or down. I couldn't turn my head, either, and I could barely walk. Basically, I couldn't do anything at that point. It would be two weeks before I could even take them out on my own, with caution and modifications. Not at all like our walks before.

My friend came to see me around that two-week mark, and she set up some agility equipment for me. I had forgotten how important this was to me. She set up weave poles and a couple of jumps so I could just stand there and send the dogs through at a distance. I'm not a distance handler, but that's just what we had to do to make it work. I couldn't even bend over to pick up a jump bar, so if they knocked a bar, I had to wait until my husband came home to fix it.

The training at home was fun, and doing agility improved my walking abilities. I also began walking my dogs in the six-acre pasture at my house. I would use a jump bar as a cane, just in case I felt unsteady. When you take the dogs in the field, they are usually crazy, but that wasn't the case when I was recovering. They walked nicely with me, never ran or darted, and I was never afraid of being knocked down. As I continued to improve, they became more and more like their usual selves. I didn't leash-walk my dogs for months, and when I did, it was short and in a controlled environment.

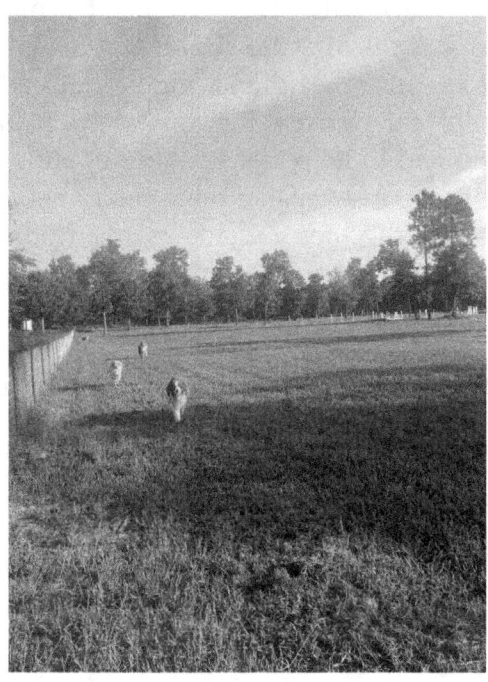

In the months before, I had been showing my dogs once a month when I would return to Ohio for work. After the accident, I could not travel until sometime in September, and even then, it was way too soon. The trip was exhausting and very difficult for me. I still couldn't bend over, do stairs, or anything like that. It was a very challenging trip.

In the yard at home, I would send the dogs through the equipment and walk beside them to get them to do small courses. Though it was probably too soon, I entered Zigzag in the trial, and I walked the course. I had someone run him a few times that fall because I still couldn't run, and I didn't want to frustrate him with walking. I continued to walk the courses until the end of

December. I wasn't allowed to run until then, so it was more like January when I actually began running.

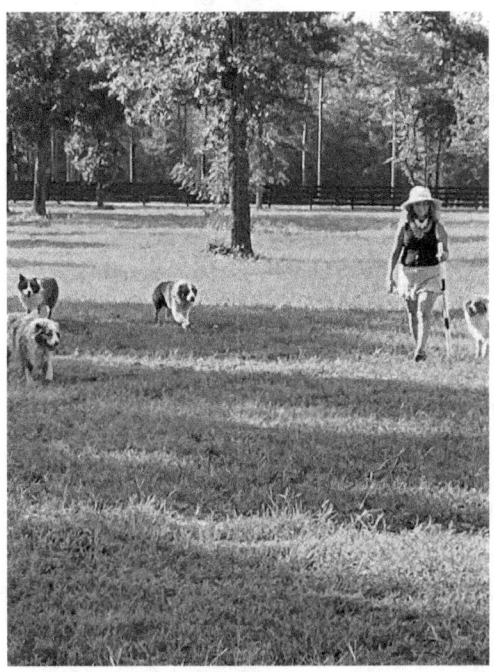

I did get one qualifying score by walking the course with my younger dog, Rip, and I came close several times with Zigzag. We could work on contact performance and obstacle commitment while I couldn't run. Even once I started running, I had to wear my brace. I know it made many people nervous, watching someone out there in a neck brace. I was concerned that I couldn't turn my head to maintain a connection and see where I was going on the course. So, my peripheral vision was essential. Sometimes, it's all I had. Soon, Zigzag and I began to get doubles and premieres, and in early 2024, we were able to qualify for the AKC Nationals!

When I think back on how far I've come in such a short time, I'm pretty happy about that. To go from standing still and being unable to pick up a jump bar to qualifying for the Nationals in a few short months was incredible. I didn't realize how much dog agility meant to me until I went through this experience.

One time, my first agility dog, Flip, injured himself and couldn't do agility, and I missed it then, too. It's the connection that you miss—the relationship. I needed that after my accident because I felt so disconnected from everyone and myself. So, standing out there and telling them to jump and weave was an amazing emotional and physical boost. It was a reason to get up in the morning and keep trying. Having the goal of making Nationals just kept pushing me to do it.

It's so nice not to have limitations now. Walking with my dogs is one of my true happy places. When I couldn't do it at all, I didn't feel like myself. Having that six-acre pasture to let them trot around with me was amazing. I could hang onto the fence and my jump bar and be completely safe with my dogs. Now, when I have a day when I'm unable to open a jar or pick something up, I just think about the little increments, the improvements that came over time, and then I take a breath and realize it will all come together if I just give it time.

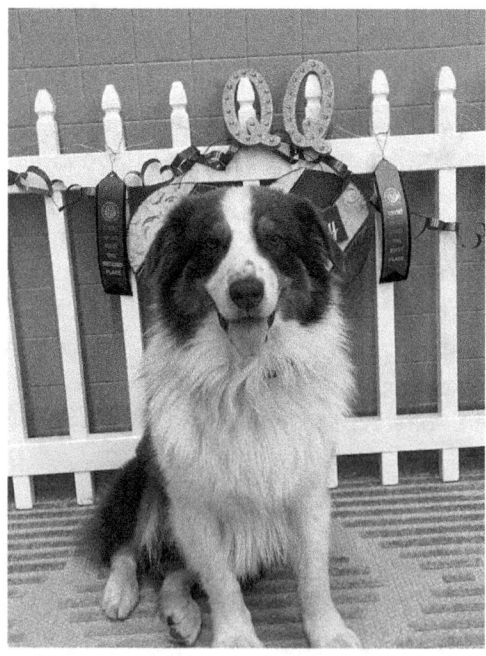

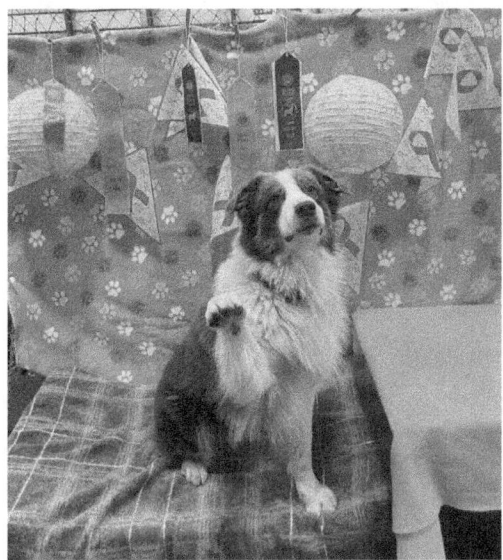

Gratitude

I knew from the beginning that my physical recovery was something that I could control; something I had been trained to do. What I couldn't control, though, was how others supported me in that climb, and I was pleasantly surprised by what happened. Even though many of my friends and clients do not live here in Aiken, they supported me by calling, texting, and messaging me and sending me grocery and restaurant gift cards to help make up for some of my lost income. Their encouraging words were so helpful! The emotional support that I received from clients and friends I've known my entire life was wonderful, but I was surprised by all the support from people I barely knew.

I hadn't lived in Aiken very long when the accident happened, so when I was in pain or feeling incapable, feeling like things would never improve, I thought I would be alone. But there was always someone at my window to drop off a protein shake, a salad, or dinner or just to say hi. Sometimes people would ask me a question about something that was going on or just text me a joke. They would drop off shirts that were easier for me to put on, like button-ups, since I couldn't pull anything over my head. Before I could fix my hair, a kind neighbor would come over to brush and braid it for me. You can't create or buy that kind of support. You just have to be lucky enough to have it.

My amazing friends helped get me to work when I started working again, which I did way earlier than I should have. Plus, they helped me with some of the more physically challenging parts of my job. I walked them through those tasks as if I were training them. They rode my horses and walked my dogs. They even set my agility course. Some very generous people helped with a meal train, and one kind soul paid for somatic therapy, which helped me get past the trauma. I wanted to recover and not only become physically as strong as I was before—which I'm still working toward—but mentally stronger too.

To think that people took time out of their lives to try to make mine a little more pleasant was so moving to me, and I am eternally grateful for that. In the moments when I felt like I had nothing to give or contribute, like I was taking instead of giving, someone would remind me of how I had helped their dog or horse. It made me feel like I wasn't taking, like I was part of the community.

The accident gave me a glimpse of something I would never have known existed. Whether it was my best friend from when I was two, a client I had for years, or a person I'd met on the street who just happened to give me an encouraging smile, I wanted to thank each and every person who supported me. Whether they wrote a note on Facebook, sent messages or letters, called, texted, or whatever, every single one of those acts of kindness made my recovery possible. Without my community of supporters, both in Aiken and around the world, I would not have recovered as well as I have. All the encouragement and support made the difficult times easier. Sometimes people can amaze you!

One of my friends went above and beyond what I ever could have expected, and I wanted to mention her contributions here. During my recovery, even something as simple as getting dressed proved to be a challenge. My friend helped me find bras that I could put on by myself. Regular bras fasten on the back, and I couldn't get my hands behind my back, and I didn't have the strength in my hands to put them on. Only a friend thinks of things like that. This is the same friend who brought me to Africa for the first time, and I'm so grateful to her for all she did for me.

When I went to Africa, I visited Tanzania, and it was a weird feeling. I felt like I was supposed to be back there. I loved being back there! But the travel made me realize that this was as early as I could've possibly done it. We were camping, and the flights were long. The vehicles we took out on the game drives were bumpy, and the horses we rode were not as well-trained as the ones at home. The walks were also long and sometimes dicey. But I loved being there. I felt like I needed to go back. I had some purpose in being there.

I had some fantastic new experiences on the trip. I saw a cheetah hunting and another one with her cub. I went in a hot air balloon and saw the migration and the Serengeti from above. I saw lions and lion cubs, and we chased baboons away from a cheetah cub to try to save its life (hopefully, that worked out). I saw a black rhino in the Serengeti from a distance, and we went to another sanctuary in the north where they have a black rhino breeding facility, and I got to see more. Seeing their conservation efforts was uplifting.

The black rhino was the animal that first brought me to Africa, when I went to a black rhino facility in Kenya. As I mentioned at the beginning of the book, my zookeeper friend had won a trip by raising money for that facility, and they brought me along, which began my absolute obsession with Africa. I have a special affinity for these majestic creatures, so seeing them again nearly thirty years later felt amazing. I'm grateful they're still here, and I'm hopeful I can do more to help ensure they remain in our world.

At night, I went to a Maasai village when they were having a ceremony and joined in as they danced. They were very welcoming, as always, and they're always delighted to share their culture and beliefs. This particular ceremony was for a girl who had been married since 2016. Up until that night, the husband had eaten with his mother, and the girl had eaten with her friends. She was not allowed to cook or eat with him. I don't have any interest in cooking, and quite honestly, if someone told me I didn't have to cook, I'd be thrilled. But I don't live in a culture where that's an issue. The girl seemed very excited about the ceremony, and I was happy to be able to participate in it.

I danced on the women's side. They put a beaded collar around my neck and truly embraced me in their tribe. I have been with the Maasai several times before, but every time I get to be with them, I feel honored to have the experience. It's quite a different culture, and, amazingly, it has withstood the pressures of time.

We also visited a waterfall in the village, where I was nearly swept away. My friend had slid down the rocks, and as I laughed at her, I too slid down and crashed right into her. The water we had to walk through was above my waist. It was really fun.

Another amazing thing we got to do on this trip was visit the protected area where the Maasai live. You have to ask for permission to be there since the area is heavily poached. We actually saw some fires that had been lit by poachers. The animals were very skittish. If they're in the Serengeti, they know they're safe, but in the protected areas, they're not. We saw giraffes, zebras, wildebeest, and elephants, and it was amazing to see them out in the wild. The wildlife parks are small, unlike the Serengeti, which is half the size of Delaware, and it's interesting to see the animals trying to get through the parks safely.

After that, I visited a horse I had met and worked with before. He was much older by that point and had been leased out, so he was not in the best shape. But he remembered me, and I was honored by that. I worked on him, and when I returned to see him a couple of days later, he came up, nuzzled me, and wanted me to work on him again. These are the little things that make my job so special—when you're able to make a difference and the animal understands and appreciates it. I am blessed to have done that. Unfortunately, just a couple of days later, he had to be put down. This made me very sad, but I was grateful that I had given him some comfort at the end of his life and that I got to see him one more time. Unless you're an animal person, you probably don't understand that animals do remember you and that the relationship with them goes beyond words.

I wish I had some magical ending to my story, like I went on to do something amazing, but I don't. At least, not yet. The amazing thing is that I survived! Who knows what the future holds? I don't ever want to stop massaging dogs and horses. I love it so much, and through this work, I've had the opportunity to meet some amazing animals and see some incredible relationships between the animals and their human companions. It's incredible to hear the stories about how they found each other, how the animal has transformed them, or how they have transformed the animal. I always want that to be a part of what I do.

That said, I would love to do something more—write a book (check!), have a podcast, and maybe become a motivational speaker, mentor, and philanthropist. I want to get more into dog training, too, and perhaps work for a nonprofit. My options are limited, of course, because of my eyesight. Scratch that—they're not limited, just different. What I'm looking for isn't something you find on job boards. Most likely, it will come up organically through a conversation or casual meeting. I want to do something fulfilling and exciting that gives back to others.

I'm confident that, eventually, I'll do something amazing. I want to start a nonprofit that sends money to Africa to support wildlife and the people. I often think about how I was nearly dead, and honestly, it still haunts me. I know that's how it'll be for a while.

That said, I can't wait to see what the future has in store for me.

As I reached the end of my recovery from the accident, I realized that Cake and I were recovering at the same time. When I was able to free lunge her and hand walk her, I thought I was doing something for *her*; I didn't realize at the time that she was doing something for *me*, as well. Our relationship has always been about give-and-take for both of us, so helping her get better and stronger helped me get better and stronger. When we both were able to ride together, it was incredible. The first time I went to a show with her sound and happy, I was sound and happy, too. It was incredible to jump her around again in a Hunter show ring. That meant we were both healed. I'm sure there will be ups and downs along the road for both of us in the future, but we made it this far, so I know we can take them on.

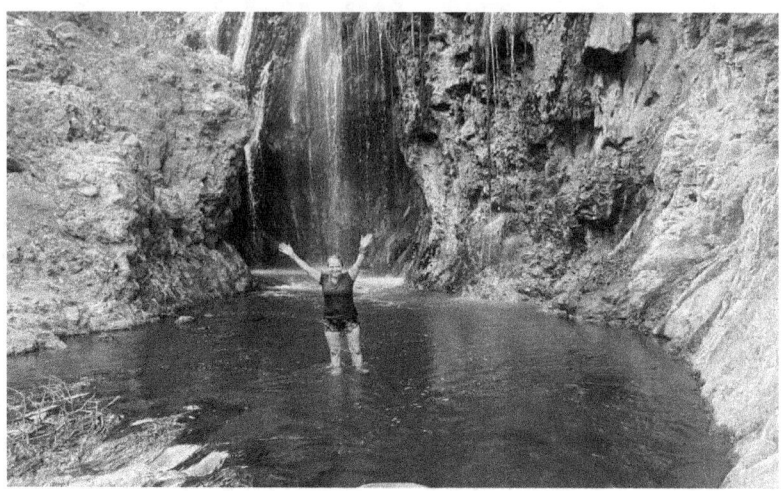

Facebook Post 5/10/2024

Today, I am having a grateful day. You guys have been there with me throughout my entire accident, and I have often told you about how hard it's been. Well, now you get to hear how amazing it is for me to be able to lift anything I want. Lol, that's a big deal for me, but to be able to take Chocolate Cake after her surgery and after mine, and jump around in my field where my accident was and be happy is the best thing ever! I love this horse, and again, I want to thank you for all your support throughout this whole thing. It's good that it's over.

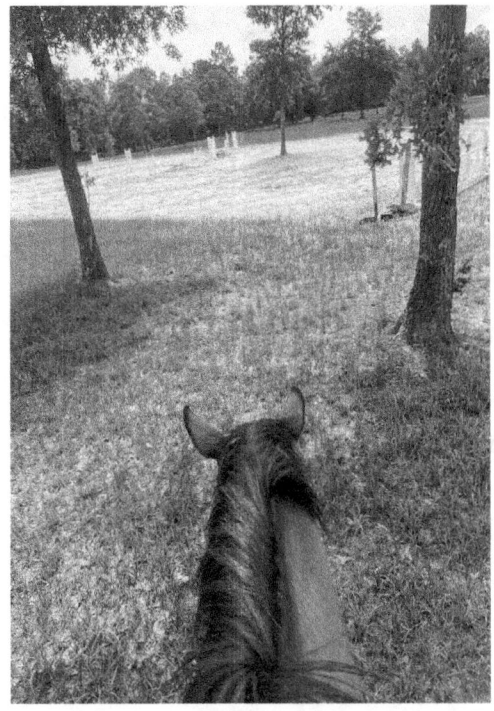

About the Author

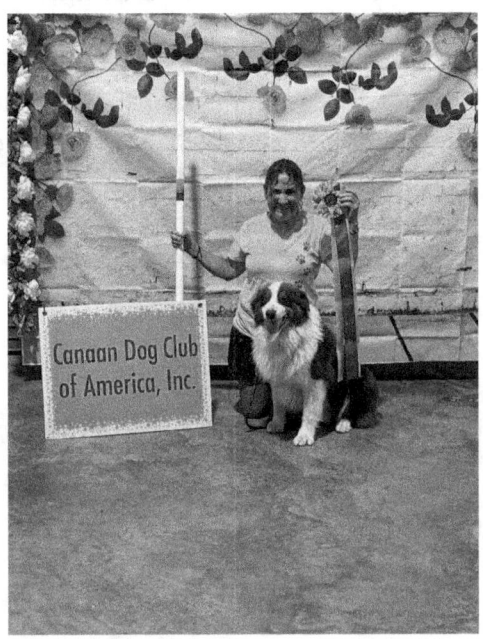

Canaan Dog Club of America, Inc.

Maria K. McManus Duthie is the owner of Annisage, as a highly recommended canine and equine massage therapist. With over twenty-five years of behavioral and anatomical knowledge, she works to promote healthier animals from the inside out.

Maria completed her massage training through the Optissage program in Circleville, Ohio. She also studied animal science at the University of Florida and exotic animal management at the Santa Fe Teaching Zoo, along with earlier studies at Indiana University. She has owned horses for over twenty-five years and has worked as a stable manager, groomer, trainer, and exercise rider in several stables with various disciplines.

As a zookeeper for four years, Maria wrote several papers on behavioral enrichment. While in this position, she saw firsthand the correlation between physical pain and behavioral problems.

She then began to study several forms of healing touch and behavior modification. In addition to exotics, Maria has studied dog, cat, and horse behavior. Combining behavioral knowledge, anatomical knowledge, and massage techniques, she is able to work with animals on several levels.

Annisage is a complete animal wellness service for equine, canine, feline, and exotic animals. The focus on massage and bodywork promotes healthier animals, from house pets to competitors.

www.ingramcontent.com/pod-product-compliance
Lightning Source LLC
Chambersburg PA
CBHW071208120626
46546CB00006B/2474